A CURIOUS MAN'S
Guide to
Urology

Sex, Stones, Prostate Woes, and More!

DR. STEPHEN F LIEBERMAN, M.D.

A CURIOUS MAN'S GUIDE TO UROLOGY

Sex, Stones,Prostate Woes, and More!

Veru Montanum Press

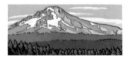

Portland, Oregon, USA 97035

Book cover design by: Susan Bein
Illustrations by: Mogumash
Book layout design by: Saqib_arshad

Printed in the United States of America

stephenliebermanmd.com

For my mom and dad,

Bernice and Eddie

&

Luis E. Halpert M.D.

What other's are saying about
The Curious Man's Guide to Urology

"Dr Steve Lieberman provides straight, unbiased information for common men's conditions that is easy to read and understand. It's a great resource I recommend to my patients and colleagues."

- Ron Loo, M.D. Chief Emeritus Southern California Kaiser Permanente Medical Group.

"This is a remarkably lucid, beautifully written discussion of all aspects of male urological medical and emotional topics. Anyone reading this book will be well-informed, empowered, and able to engage in a meaningful discussion with his urologist. Dr. Lieberman explains issues in a tremendously helpful, clear manner, with equal amounts of knowledge, sound advice and charm."

—Roger Porter, Professor of English, Emeritus, Reed College

"Looking for a good read on some delicate, sometimes embarrassing topics? You've found it!"

—John M. Barry, M.D., Professor of Urology, Professor of Surgery, Division of Abdominal Organ Transplantation, Oregon Health & Science University, Portland, Oregon

"Dr. Lieberman is one of the finest clinicians and passionate teachers about everything related to urology. Whether you are a patient or clinician, this book is packed with useful information about the urinary system. You'll get easy-to-understand answers to the questions you were too afraid to ask. His practical and insightful pearls taught in a conversational style will keep you engaged."

—Jill Einstein, M.D., Senior Director, MAVEN Project

TABLE OF CONTENTS

INTRODUCTION

If you're reading this book, chances are you or someone you love has a health problem related to the urinary tract system. There is a lot going on in that system which is comprised of our kidneys, adrenal glands, ureter, bladder and urethra. For men this includes the scrotum, prostate and penis. If you're like most men, you might think about your penis a fair amount, but for most of us, we don't think much about the rest of our urinary tract until something goes wrong—then we want medical help, and we want it quickly. That's because our health—and our peace of mind—depends on having an efficient fluid waste system for everything we eat and drink. When our plumbing gets stopped up, so to speak, something is wrong.

I'm the guy many came to when they want to know what it is that's wrong, and how to make it right. I practiced general urology at Kaiser Permanente in Portland, Oregon for 31 years. I was Chief of the Urology Department for 27 of those 31 years. I witnessed remarkable changes in the profession over those decades as advances in medicine and new technological innovations provided a range of options for patients, often options which saved their lives when just a few years before their lives would have been cut short. Yet with our rapidly expanding medical knowledge, technologies and medicines, come not only choices for our patients, but decisions to be made. For every option, there are considerations, and not everything in medicine is certain. What might work for one patient may not work for another. What one patient can adapt to, another may be unable or unwilling to consider. Whether it's medication, surgery, diet, radiation, or time—the wait and see approach—it's important that you be as informed as possible so that you can make the decision that's best for you—and hopefully, in agreement with your physician.

I've written this book to help you to do just that—to understand your body, particularly your urinary and genital system, better. What does it means when one or more components of your urinary tract system aren't working properly? What are your options to make it better? What are the risks of the treatment? Knowing these things will enable you to engage in shared decision making—the foundation of a patient centered approach to medicine, and the underlying concept of this book.

Shared decision making is a popular concept in contemporary medicine that refers to a decision making process in which both the patient and his or her physician work together in designing the best plan of care for the patient. This process departs from the traditional top-down model of medical care where the physician tells the patient what s/he needs to do. In shared decision making, the patient's values, cultural background, goals and concerns are considered. The patient (and family) are active participants throughout diagnosis and treatment. By "active participant," I don't just mean the patient shows up for tests and procedures—of course you're going to participate in your own health care by showing up. What I mean is you are armed with information about the procedures, the tests, the medications, and your health conditions, so that the decisions you make are informed ones. By knowing more about your health condition, by being aware of the medications, technologies, procedures and treatment plans available to you, and their risks and benefits, you are better able to ask questions, share your concerns, and work constructively with your physician in treating your health conditions.

We weren't taught shared decision making in medical school when I was a medical student 40 years ago. In those days, such an approach would come under the umbrella of "the art of medicine" or "bedside manner." Some might call it physician empathy. Only recently has the value of patient centered medicine and shared decision making been recognized by the medical profession. Early in my career, however, many of us intuitively appreciated how important it is that our patients be as informed and engaged in their treatment as possible. In more recent years, the increased focus on shared decision making or patient engagement has enhanced and improved the overall care of the patient.

Shared decision making is not for everyone, nor does it apply to every situation or every medical decision. There are some patients who are more comfortable with a paternalistic model. These patients come to me saying something along the lines of, "Just fix it doc, do what you think is best." And there are some situations (emergencies for example) in which there is only one way of taking care of the immediate problem, regardless of what the patient might prefer. In these cases, a decision can't be contemplated or delayed without putting the patient's life or organ at risk.

Shared decision making is best suited for complicated illnesses and treatments. Shared decision making is beneficial and well suited for those problems that aren't "fixed" with one solution but will instead require a series of treatments, or for those problems that do not have a single answer but have instead, multiple options, each with risks and benefits.

The treatment of prostate cancer is a good example in which there are many treatment options (surgery, radiation, or active surveillance for localized cancer). They can all produce good long-term outcomes, with only slight differences in "cure rates," but each treatment differs in terms of potential complications and side effects. There is no "one size fits all" treatment for prostate cancer, so if you are suffering from prostate cancer, you will want to know as much as possible about your options, and about your specific cancer.

That's why I've written this book—to give you the basic knowledge of your urinary tract system, the most common problems that urologists treat, and the most effective and up to date treatment options. You're unlikely to need or want to read this book in its entirety, although I encourage you to do so. By having a solid understanding of your entire urinary tract system, you will better understand how the differing components of that system work together. At the very least, I urge you to begin the book by reading Chapter 1, "Your Body's Plumbing." That chapter is a concise overview of how we're plumbed, and what happens when our plumbing is damaged. Other chapters are organized around various ailments (cancers of urinary tract organs, stones, blood in the urine, infections) or other pertinent concerns (circumcision, vasectomy, urinary tract trauma, and emergencies).

In Chapter 2, "Mysteries of the Foreskin and Circumcision," I discuss not only the removal of the foreskin as a medical procedure, but the cultural origins of what as far as I know is the only near universal form of bodily modification for males. (Piercings and tattoos are other universal forms of bodily modification, but done for cosmetic and social, not health, purposes, and are not exclusive to men, whereas female circumcision is far from universal, and is done for social, not health reasons.)

Chapter 3, "I'm Peeing Blood," focuses on the causes of blood in the urine. Because blood in the urine is often a sign of other problems, such as kidney stones or bladder cancer, you may come to this chapter not knowing what is wrong, or you may already know and find that this chapter, along with one or more others specific to your health problem, are valuable reading.

Chapter 4, "Urinary Tract Infections" discusses a relatively rare problem for men, but if you have a UTI, you want to address it. In this chapter, I discuss a number of different UTI's, including cystitis, prostatitis, pyelonephritis, bacteriuria, and epididymitis, how each is diagnosed, and how each is treated.

Sometimes the problem isn't blood in your pee or painful urination, but the inability to pee at all. If that is your concern, in Chapter 5, "Can't Pee, See Me," I cover the reasons why you may be blocked, including one of the most common reasons—Benign Prostate Hyperplasia—and what your options are to resolve this annoying and potentially dangerous problem

One of the most common questions I get asked is whether a man should get his PSA checked. Chapter 6, "Should I Get a PSA," answers that question and more about the Prostate Specific Antigen test that can reveal early stages of prostate cancer.

Chapter 7, "Prostate Cancer," takes a close look at different types of prostate cancer, how to treat it, and how to live with it.

Chapter 8, "Your Scrotum and Testicles," is on just that—your balls, which hang in your ball sac, and for all the pleasure they may bring you, they occasionally bring you pain. In that chapter, I discuss not only testicular cancer, but testicular torsion, sperm production, pain, swelling, inguinal hernia, infection and other things that go wrong with your testicles and scrotum.

In Chapter 9, "Bladder Cancer," I discuss this relatively common, but increasingly curable disease, the many forms of bladder cancer, your treatment options if you are diagnosed with it, and your quality of life should you have to have your bladder removed; (I assure you, a cystectomy, the surgical removal of the bladder, does not by any means suggest your quality of life will suffer in any meaningful way, but it may well save your life).

In Chapter 10, I turn to the kidneys in the chapter titled, "Everybody Must Get Stones." If you've ever had a kidney stone, you know it can produce indescribable pain. Kidney stone pain or renal colic has been compared to childbirth. It may take hours, if not days, to pass those cursed stones. For some people, kidney stones are a frequent occurrence, while for others, they appear only once never to return— or they may not cause renal colic at all but present as a UTI or blood in the urine. In this chapter I dispel the many myths you may see on the internet about stones, and explain just how diet, heredity, and other factors lead to different types of stones and how to hopefully prevent them from recurring.

Kidney masses are discussed in Chapter 11, "Kidney Tumors, Cysts, and Masses," I discuss what those lumps and tumors might be, which ones are benign, which are malignant, and depending on the diagnosis, what your treatment options are. The good news is, we've never before had the remarkable technologies to treat cancerous kidneys. You'll learn which kidney masses are benign and don't need treatment. But, if the tumor is cancer, I'll present the most effective technologies now available.

Chapter 12, "Erectile Dysfunction," I explain the many reasons this common, but usually unwelcome, disorder affects many men, how to avoid it, and what to watch for when taking ED medications.

Chapter 13 is on "Vasectomies." If you are planning or thinking of getting a vasectomy, congratulations! It means you're probably in good health. But that doesn't mean the procedure won't come with significant concerns, ambivalence, minor discomfort, or just a lot of questions. In this chapter I do my best to answer the most common among these concerns and questions, as well as discuss reversing the procedure should your circumstances and/or views on having children change.

Finally, Chapter 14 focuses on "Emergencies and Traumas." These are the sorts of things that you probably won't have time to look up beforehand, but may well have questions about after you've received treatment, such as injuries, unexpected and life-endangering medical emergencies, or complications related to prior procedures. This is the only chapter where shared decision making is of less concern because the main concern is saving your life and/or addressing the issue as quickly as possible is paramount. I hope you never have need of this chapter, but should you have such an emergency or trauma, I want you to rest assured your concerns are answered.

Regardless of whether you read the whole book or only the chapters of most concern to you, I encourage you to read the Conclusion, where I summarize the importance of good urinary tract health and what you can do to ensure yours is the best it can be. One of those things is knowing how to work with your physician and medical team to remain an informed and engaged participant in your treatment from the very first day you walk into your physician's office. To help you stay engaged, I've included a list of resources, with a link to my website where you can stay up-to-date on the most recent advances in urological care, as well as a Glossary for those terms you might forget after my initial definition.

In closing, a few words on my own personal bias. We live in an amazing age, where information on any topic imaginable is available to almost anyone with a laptop and access to Google. But with that information comes a great deal of bias, misinformation, and disinformation - BMD. As a patient, you may find yourself on your own as you scrounge the internet for information on your health, finding millions of hits that do more to scare and confuse you than inform you. We've seen this confusion most recently with the COVID pandemic, where we've been bombarded with conflicting information. "Where did it start, in the open market or the lab in Wuhan?" "Was it intentional germ warfare, an accident, or a natural mutation?" "It's just like the flu, no big deal!" "It will kill you if you get it!" "Masks don't work, masks make you sick, masks save your life." "What about Ivermectin?" "Are the vaccines safe? How many do we need? Will they make you infertile? Will they make you magnetic?" This "BMD" has resulted in far too many illnesses, injuries and deaths, not just in the United States, but throughout the world.

There is bias, misinformation and disinformation in urology, as well. In writing this book, I want to be clear that I will declare my bias and try to be transparent about it (eg early detection of prostate cancer, or evaluation of microscopic blood in the urine). In those cases, I present alternative views and provide the data and reasoning that support my positions. There are many areas of medicine that are not black or white, with no single absolute right answer. Medicine is an art as much as a science, and as physicians we must draw conclusions and make decisions involving a number of differing factors. That's why shared decision making is so important—the more your physician knows about you and your needs, the more likely the decisions you make together will be the best decisions for you. By sharing my own biases in areas where I know there are differing views, the better equipped you'll be to draw your own conclusions.

But before you can draw any informed conclusions about your urological health, you need to know something about your own plumbing. So pour yourself a hot or cold drink, turn the page, and let me tell you how that drink will wind up in the toilet in a few hours.

CHAPTER 1

Your Body's Plumbing

If you think of your central nervous system as your body's electrical system and your gastrointestinal system as your body's waste management system, then it makes sense to think of your genitourinary system as your body's plumbing system. Why think of something as complex as the human body in such simplified abstract terms? Because thinking of your body in this way makes it easier to understand. And because for all the wonders of the human body, it's basically a mechanical system of inter-related parts that function interdependently to keep you alive—until, of course, one or more of those parts breaks down. That's when you call someone like me, a urologist, to diagnose the problem and propose one or more ways to fix it.

Understanding your body's plumbing may help you to make decisions about your medical care. If you possess an appreciation of your anatomy and physiology, the decisions you make with your doctor will be more informed than the typical, "Oh, just do whatever you think is right, Doc, and get it over with," response. We doctors appreciate a patient who understands how his body is put together and takes an active role in his treatment. So how is your genitourinary system put together? Let's start with the basic parts, sort of like figuring out what all these parts are to the Ikea product you just bought and have to put together.

There are eight basic parts we're going to talk about in this book: the adrenal glands, the kidneys, the ureter, bladder, prostate, urethra, penis and scrotum and testes. Whether you're having a problem urinating, suffer from erectile dysfunction, infertility, kidney stones or a related cancer, one or more of these organs or parts will be affected. So let's take a look at where they are and what they do.

Remember that glass of water (or whiskey) I suggested you pour at the end of the Introduction. Well now's the time to drink it. Take a good long sip of your water, or a more modest sip of your whiskey, and feel it pass your lips, wet your tongue and glide down your throat until you can no longer feel it. Now that you can no longer feel it, what's it doing in the darkness of your inner body?

As that liquid flows down your throat, it already starts its work hydrating your mouth, esophagus, and stomach. As it does so, your brain receives signals that you are becoming hydrated. That's why after only a few sips of water, you might feel as if you've had enough— even if you really do need more. But if your brain didn't tell you you'd had enough early on, you'd keep drinking, potentially consuming too much by the time your brain was happy. It's going to take time for all the cells in your body to become hydrated by that drink, which is why your brain wants you to drink slowly—and steadily—throughout the day.

Your esophagus is a tube that connects your mouth to your stomach. As you fill your stomach with the fluid you are drinking, the fluid is transported to your small intestines, where it is absorbed and then enters your bloodstream.

Fluid absorption starts once the the liquid reaches the small intestines (small intestines are about 20 feet long and stuffed inside of you like one of those collapsible hoses shoved inside a garbage bag at the end of the summer). The large intestines are wrapped around the small intestines like a frame. Fluid/water absorption continues in the large intestine and it's here in the that the cells in your body get the most benefit (or cost) from whatever it is that you're drinking, as the liquid reaches your bloodstream and hydrates your organs, tissues, muscles and cells.

Once your body has absorbed all the water it needs, it needs to get rid of what it doesn't need. There are four ways your body eliminates water—through your large intestines, in the form of feces; through your mouth, in the form of saliva; through your skin in the form of sweat; and through your kidneys in the form of urine. It's this last process we're concerned with here, as the water now in your bloodstream reaches your urinary tract.

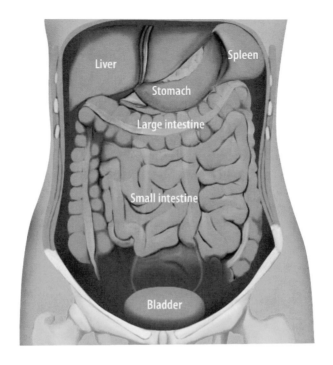

Intra-peritoneal Anatomy

The urinary tract starts in the abdomen in the space called the retroperitoneum. Retro means "behind," so the retroperitoneum refers to the space behind the peritoneum. The peritoneum is the abdominal space where your guts (stomach, small intestine, and parts of the large intestine), liver, and spleen reside. Also housed in the retroperitoneum are lymph channels running alongside your blood vessels and carrying lymph fluid, which is a byproduct of the filtration of blood returning to the heart. Situated along the course of the lymph channel are lymph glands. These lymph glands filter the lymph fluid. These lymph glands and channels become important if cancer invades the bladder, prostate, kidneys, testes or penis, because if the cancer invades them, the cancer can spread to the pelvis and throughout the retro-peritoneum. For this reason, certain cancer surgeries call for the removal of these glands and channels.

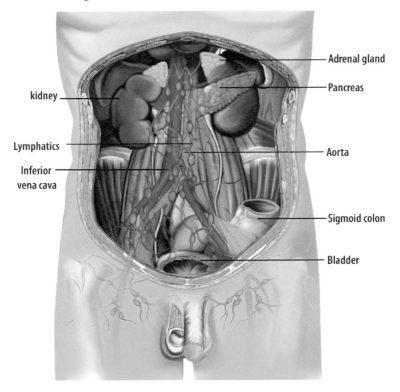

kidney

Lymphatics

Inferior
vena cava

Adrenal gland

Pancreas

Aorta

Sigmoid colon

Bladder

Retroperitoneal Anatomy

The urinary tract itself consists of the kidneys, ureters, bladder, prostate, and urethra. Your kidneys are two bean-shaped organs, each about the size of two fists pressed together. Your two largest blood vessels, the aorta and vena cava, supply blood to the kidneys through the renal arteries, and take blood back to the vena cava and eventually the heart via the renal veins. On top of your kidneys are your adrenal glands, which are shaped liked large fortune cookies or Jewish haman-taschen cookies. These glands produce three important hormones—steroids, adrenaline, and noradrenaline—which regulate your heartbeat, blood pressure, and serve other critical functions. Water reaches your kidneys through the bloodstream, just as it reaches other organs in your body. Without water reaching every organ, muscle and tissue, we'd be mummified inside. But unlike other organs in your body, the kidneys play a particularly important role in water regulation. The kidneys play an important role in maintaining hydration and water balance and hydration throughout your body. Your kidneys also filter your blood and regulate vitamins, minerals, enzymes and hormones needed to stay alive, such as renin, an enzyme to regulate your blood pressure and erythropoietin, a hormone which helps produce red blood cells. The kidneys also activate Vitamin D. No wonder you're in trouble if you have a problem with your kidneys! So how do they do all this?

Well, to simplify the process, once the water you've consumed is absorbed into your bloodstream, it reaches your kidneys by series of arteries, which enter the kidneys into a vast network of microscopic blood vessels (arterioles). These tiny vessels are intwined with approximately two million tiny nephrons, which form a powerful network of detectors and filters. These nephrons identify anything the body needs, which is then reabsorbed by the nephron. Anything your body doesn't need, like urea (a byproduct of proteins) as well as any excess water your body doesn't need, is eliminated by the nephron. The combination of water and waste products that you don't need is urine.

Chemicals, salts (such as sodium and potassium), toxic waste, amino acids, vitamins, glucose, water, and other elements are regulated by the nephrons. Some of these substances, compounds, and electrolytes are filtered and excreted in the urine, while some are reabsorbed and put back into the bloodstream. Others are "regulated" so that just the right amount winds up back in the bloodstream. The nephrons add excess water to the things your body doesn't need to make urine. The more excess water you have in your body, the more hydrated you are, the more light-colored the urine will be. In contrast, the less hydrated you are, the more cloudy or dark your urine will be, given there is less water to dilute the waste products your kidneys are trying to eliminate.

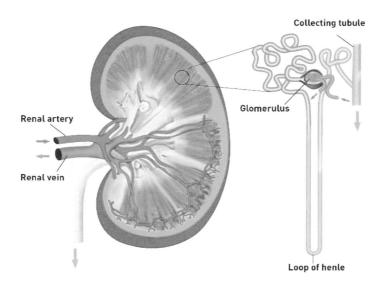

Kidney (L) and glomerulus (R) anatomy

That water and waste (now urine) travel through the ureters, which are foot long tubes about the diameter of a pencil that connect each kidney to the bladder. The inner lumen of each ureter is about 2 mm. (a common knitting needle and the tip of a new crayon are 2 mm, or 0.08 inches)

Your bladder is a hollow muscle-walled organ that rests on your pelvic floor and temporarily stores your urine. It has three openings— the two openings where the ureters drain urine into the bladder, and the urethra (in males the beginning of the prostate where the bladder joins the prostate, also known as the prostatic urethra), where the urine leaves the bladder. The bladder is passively stretched until it reaches full capacity. When your bladder is full, it sends a message up the spinal cord and to the brain telling your brain that your bladder is full and you need to pee. When that happens, as soon as you have un-zipped your pants and pulled them down, your brain turns off the in-hibitory fibers that travel down the spinal cord, the valves open, your bladder muscle contracts, and your pee is released, much to your re-lief.

The urethra, is ten to twelve inches long, beginning where the bladder joins the prostate and ending at the tip of the penis. A woman's urethra is two inches long. The discrepancy between male and female urethras explains why women get more bladder infections than men. The bacteria have a much shorter distance to travel.

The urethra goes through the prostate. Think of putting a straw (urethra) through an orange (prostate). At the end of the prostate, the urethra goes though the pelvic floor muscle (also called the external sphincter). This muscle can be contracted and relaxed voluntarily. This is what's happening if you voluntarily shut off and restart your stream during urination. The straw (urethra) continues through the length of the penis, ending at the tip (urethral meatus).

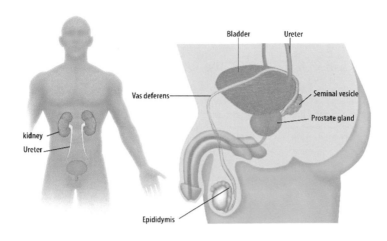

Male Genito-Urinary Anatomy

The penis is made up of three tubes—the urethra, and the two erectile tubes called the corpora cavernous. In an erect penis, the corporal bodies are like blood filled sponges in a tough fibrous casing. When the fun is over, the sponges empty and the penis becomes flaccid (more about this in a sec) Peyronie's disease is abnormal scar tissue that occurs in the tough casing (tunica albuginea).The urethra is underneath both erectile chambers. It's what you pee through as you empty your bladder. Semen also comes (no pun intended) though the urethra.

Let's say you've poured yourself a nice glass of wine and now you lift your eyes from the page to the face of a nearby partner, and before you know it, your penis is coming alive and the last thing you're thinking about is your plumbing. What's happening down there? Well tell your partner to hold on, because now we're going to talk about sex and fertility.

It was once thought that the penis became erect as a result of air, as if the penis were some sort of balloon. But one of the first to dispel us of this mistaken perception was none other than one of our earliest anatomists, Leonardo da Vinci, the painter of the enigmatic Mona Lisa. Leonardo wrote one of the earliest treatises on the penis, after watching dissections of hanged men—a common practice of Renaissance artists as the bodies of executed criminals were used to teach anatomy to medical students and painters of the human body.

Leonardo was struck by the erections he noted in these cadavers, and that in each case, the erections were filled with blood—not air.

> I have seen … dead men who have the member erected, for many die thus, especially those hanged. Of these [penises] I have seen the anatomy, all of them having great density and hardness, and being quite filled by a large quantity of blood. … If an adversary says wind caused this enlargement and hardness, as in a ball with which one plays, I say such wind gives neither weight nor density. … Besides, one sees that an erect penis has a red glans, which is the sign of the inflow of blood; and when it is not erect, this glans has a whitish surface.[i]

The corpora cavernosa are the erectile bodies of your penis. They act like a sponge. When your penis is flaccid, there's just enough blood in them to keep the tissue viable. When the two sponges fill with blood, however, your penis stiffens. If you have poor blood flow to the penis, such as from severe hardening of the arteries (atherosclerosis), you may have trouble getting or keeping an erection. For an erection to happen, your penis needs blood, as well as input from nerves and, importantly, testosterone which is the main male hormone in men.

While that erection may be altered by your brain and emotions, you need testosterone made by the testes in the scrotum to complete the package.

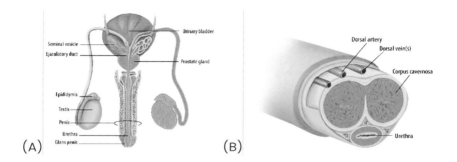

(A) Male Reproductive and Lower Urinary Tract
(B) Cross section Anatomy of the Penis

The scrotum contains the testes, epididymis, and the first part of the vas deferens. The testes are spongy organs too, also covered by a tough layer. The testes produce sperm and testosterone. How does sperm get from the testicle to the urethra to become part of the ejaculate exiting the penis? After going through a series of tubes and ducts, it passes into the vas deferens. The spermatozoa are made by cells in the testes, and as they mature, they journey via the semineferous tubules toward small straight tubes at the top back part of the testes called ductuli efferentes. The ductuli efferentes fuse together at the back of each testes, forming the epididymis, which is essentially one long tube about the length of a caterpillar, The one thin long tube (8 feet if you stretch it out) is tightly coiled in each epididymis. Each vas deferens leaves the scrotum and courses alongside the pubic bone where they enter the groin. They then enter the retroperitoneum and circle back toward the space between the bladder and prostate (on top) and the rectum (below). The two vas join two semen glands called seminal vesicles to form the ejaculatory ducts. This seminal fluid is comprised of 90% semen, and ten percent sperm and prostate secretions. These prostatic secretions nourish and protect the sperm and enhance fertility.

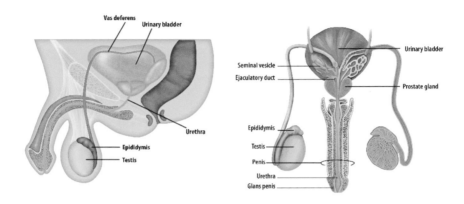

Male Reproductive and Lower Urinary Tract

You may or may not be familiar with your prostate. It's a gland about the size of a golf ball (in a 20-30 year old) and found on the lower side of your bladder (toward your feet) and above your rectum. The prostate produces an alkaline substance that mixes with your semen and neutralizes the acidity of the vaginal tract, thus protecting sperm and enhancing reproduction.

The prostate also acts as a mechanism that plays a part during urination and ejaculation. During ejaculation, the muscles surrounding the ejaculatory ducts, seminal vesicles, and prostate rhythmically contract, while simultaneously the internal sphincter (the smooth muscle part of the bladder and prostate where the bladder connects to the prostate) contracts thereby closing the connection between bladder and prostatic urethra. The semen is then expelled through the penis as chants of, "Oh God" or "Hallelujah," are heard throughout the neighborhood. If the internal sphincter is relaxed or "paralyzed" from medication (Flomax for example, given for BPH), the internal sphincter (bladder neck) stays open during ejaculation and the semen goes backward into the bladder. This is called "retrograde ejaculation".

https://www.dropbox.com/s/2fe69huyg7wlb0h/Prostate%20anatomy%20video.mov?dl=0

Conclusion

Of course, this whole description of your body's plumbing is an overly simplified thumbnail sketch of all that's going on inside but provides you with a basic understanding of the urological network that we urologists do our best to keep in good working order. By understanding how your body works, you are better able to make informed decisions about your healthcare. The better you understand your anatomy and how your body functions, the better you can assess potential risks, complications, and benefits of your treatment, including the medicines prescribed to you and any surgical options.

No matter what your urologic problem or issue may be, whether a kidney stone, blood in your urine, trouble urinating, or you are considering a vasectomy, it helps to have a sense of how all your relevant body parts connect and function. In the chapters that follow, we'll look more closely at your particular concerns, where I provide more detail of your anatomy and how these various components of the urinary tract, penis and prostate function—and what it means when one or more of these parts break down.

CHAPTER 2

Mysteries of the Foreskin and Circumcision

Whether you are circumcised or not, chances are you're pretty happy with your penis. If you're uncircumcised, you're just as God made you, and if you're circumcised, you're in the company of a lot of American men. The WHO estimates that the overall male circumcision rate in the states is somewhere between 76 and 92 percent. Most Western European countries, by contrast, have rates less than 20 percent. But even these numbers mask considerable regional variation within countries. What might surprise you, however, is that less than 40% of the males throughout the world are circumcised. The question is, why are males circumcised at all, and how might being circumcised or not affect your genitourinary health today?

Circumcision is the world's oldest elective surgery, but because the procedure is so old—over 15,000 years by some estimates—we don't really know for sure when or why people began removing the foreskin of the penis. We do know circumcisions have appeared in hieroglyphs from Ancient Egypt, and in the Gospel of Luke, Christ is said to have been circumcised in a cave on the eighth day of his life, giving rise to a number of depictions of Christ's circumcision in art, including in Byzantine artworks dating from the first century A.D. Circumcision may well have become a marker not just of Jewish identity, but Christian identity, as well. Saint Paul is alleged to have discouraged the practice among Christians.

We also know that there are health benefits to circumcision, and that the practice continues to reflect religious and cultural foundations. Circumcision of males is rare among Christian Europeans. Most Jewish males are routinely circumcised as newborns across the globe and Muslim boys as early as seven days and as late as puberty, while sub-Saharan Africans practice a range of elaborate circumcision ceremonies for males, usually every seven years, though the practice is relatively rare in Southern Africa. The practice is also rare in Latin America and most Asian societies. So why is it done at all? Why not leave the foreskin alone, just as God intended?

As a urologist and a Jew, I have often wondered about this peculiar form of bodily modification. If cutting away the foreskin represents a covenant between God and the "chosen people," couldn't He have spared us male infants such pain by commanding we pierce an ear or two or tattoo the Star of David between our belly button and Mr. Happy? God could have picked the uvula—that useless appendage that hangs off the soft palate in the back of your throat. That way, to tell if someone was a "member of the tribe," so to speak, instead of pulling down your pants, you would only have to say, "Ahh."

Ahh, but it had to be the poor foreskin. One clue for why the procedure may have originated came from a friend of mine, another urologist, who was called to serve in the first Gulf War in Iraq. After his return, he told me over a beer, "You wouldn't believe how many circs I had to do. These young uncircumcised guys would be marching across the desert, sand blowing up their pants, 110 in the shade, and the sand would get between their foreskin and glans and hurt like hell!"

That simple observation was a revelation. The nomadic tribes wandering around in the desert would have suffered the same pain, discomfort and inflammation as American soldiers in the Iraqi desert—if not more so, given their loose clothing. It makes sense that they'd want to remove the foreskin, which extends from the base of the glans, or head, of the penis, and envelopes the glans when the penis is flaccid. As the penis becomes erect, the glans—the most sensitive erogenous zone of the penis and containing thousands of nerve endings—is exposed. Circumcision involves removing this foreskin at the base of the glans. By removing the foreskin permanently, sharp-edged particles of sand, as well as bacteria and other irritants or contaminants, cannot become trapped between the foreskin and glans. Consequently, it is no surprise that circumcision has a number of health benefits.

Among these benefits is that HIV infection is significantly reduced in both circumcised heterosexual and homosexual men. For this reason, the World Health Organization (WHO) recommends circumcision in order to reduce HIV infection.

Uncircumcised boys have up to ten times the urinary infections of circumcised boys. Circumcised adult males have fewer urinary tract infections, are 30% less likely to contract genital herpes, and are less likely to transmit the human papillomavirus (HPV) to their sexual partners. Female partners of circumcised males are also less likely to develop cervical cancer.

Uncircumcised men can also develop problems if they are unable to retract the foreskin, a condition known as phimosis. If phimosis is present during childhood (after 5 years old) it can be quite irritating and cause an infection in the foreskin and glans, a condition called balanoposthitis. If phimosis occurs in adulthood, however, the irritation and infection can be more serious, especially if the uncircumcised man is a diabetic, in which case infection can be quite severe. Probably of greatest concern is the fact that the presence of even a retractable foreskin increases the risk (by as much as twentyfold) to adult men of squamous cell carcinoma of the penis, whereas males circumcised as infants have virtually no penile cancer. Finally, in contrast to the benefits of circumcision, there are few, if any, benefits to not being circumcised, other than the benefit of having an unmodified, natural body, and avoiding the risk of infection or injury from a botched circumcision.

In most cases, the choice to be circumcised or not is not one that men get to make—that decision is often made at birth, when the parents decide for their infant boy whether he should have his foreskin removed. For this reason, male circumcision is increasingly gaining as much controversy as female "circumcision" (modification of the labia and/or clitoral hood). Some parents choose circumcision for religious reasons, others for the health benefits, and still others because "everybody does it." If your parents had you circumcised, there is nothing you can do at this point to reverse the procedure. But do be comforted in knowing that you are at a health advantage for having had the procedure.

But what if you weren't circumcised? Does that mean that you are at risk of penile cancer, HIV, or some other problem? Rest assured that unless you plan to wander the sandy deserts anytime soon, as long as you are able to retract your foreskin and practice good hygiene, you will probably be fine. Penile cancer is exceptionally rare, and the elevated risk of other health problems is still minimal. (Uncircumcised diabetics, however, are at increased risk of problems related to balanitis.) For many uncircumcised males, however, at some point in their teen or adult life, they may want to be circumcised, or at least consult with a urologist about whether they should do so and what to expect if they have their foreskin removed later in life.

There are many reasons why adult men request circumcision. "It's hard to keep clean," patients have told me or, "I worry about STD's." "I can't retract it." "It smells bad." "I can't get it up anymore, do you think it will help? "My wife/husband/girlfriend/boyfriend wants me to do it." I've even heard, "The dog keeps wanting to bite it!"

So if you have not been circumcised and are considering the procedure, what can you expect? With a local penile block anesthetic, circumcision in adults can be done painlessly, and avoids the risks of a general anesthetic.

The procedure typically takes about half an hour, during which the entire foreskin surrounding the head of your penis will be removed, and your foreskin will be sutured to the shaft of your penis with stitches that will dissolve and not need to be removed. You will receive local anesthesia even if the procedure was done under general so that when wake up the pain and discomfort for the first 48 hours will be tolerable. For the next few days you should only need an over-the-counter analgesic. During this period your penis will be swollen and bruised, and sex will be the last thing on your mind!

Your physician will instruct you to use ice packs for ten to twenty minutes every couple of hours during these first couple of days. It's critical that you keep the incision clean, and your dressings will have to be changed as needed according to your urologist's preferences. Some physicians will request you come to their office to have the dressings changed, while others suggest follow up appointments after one to two weeks, and again six weeks later, are standard procedure.

Your recovery will take about two to three weeks, and you may even request a week off from work because you'll be sore and uncomfortable, but the pain is relatively mild. You probably won't be able to walk for the first day, but after a day of rest, you can begin walking for short periods, gradually increasing until you can walk easily. You will need to avoid getting the incision wet, so no showering until your doctor gives you the okay. You're going to want to avoid strenuous activity during your recovery. You should be back to normal after a couple of weeks, though you'll probably need to avoid sex or masturbation for a bit longer, usually 4-6 weeks.

Although this book is for adult men, I need to say a word about uncircumcised male children. The foreskin in a boy from birth to age 5 is not meant to be retracted, because the inner layer of foreskin is adherent to the glans. By age 5, these adhesions have broken down and the foreskin can start to be gently retracted. Forcefully retracting the foreskin prior to age 5 "to keep is clean" is not only unnecessary, but it can be painful and result in inflammation, scarring and phimosis. If that happens, circumcision then becomes "medically necessary" if topical steroid cream doesn't solve the phimosis.

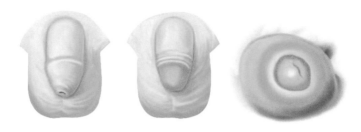

Uncircumcised Penis (L); Circumcised Penis (Center); Phimosis/Balanitis (R)

Conclusion

Circumcision is a deeply personal matter, and there are reasons for having it, and reasons for not having it. If you are looking at the overall risks and benefits, it may be better to have a circumcision. The younger you are, the easier it is. In most cases, there are no problems other than the mild pain and discomfort from the procedure. But as with any surgical procedure, there are risks. Excessive bleeding, infection, a reaction to the anesthesia, and even too much or too little foreskin removed can be problems (usually not a problem in adult circumcision when done by a urologist) One rare problem is reattachment, where the foreskin reattaches itself to the penis improperly (such as not being stitched to the shaft properly) and may require further surgery. Nonetheless, these risks are minimal, and you are unlikely to suffer any of them. When they do arise, they can usually be addressed and resolved quickly. Once you've fully recovered, whatever the reason you chose circumcision—your health, religion, social comfort or aesthetics—you are likely to find the procedure was a success.

As for whether or not to have your own sons circumcised, that is a decision to be made with care and in consultation with your partner and physician. As I've noted here, there are a number of health benefits to circumcision, and most pediatric urologists have developed a technique using a numbing cream that now makes the procedure virtually painless; some babies even sleep through the procedure. But the tradeoff is that if you choose circumcision for your infant, you are making a decision about his body that he cannot reverse. Trust yourself to make the best decision for your child and know that whether you choose to circumcise or not, your son's penis will be just fine. Isn't that what any of us want with the organ that brings us so much pleasure?

CHAPTER 3

I'm Peeing Blood!

Urologists deal with urine. We specialize in many other areas as well, but urine is our bread and butter so to speak. As you can imagine, we tell a lot of jokes about pee in the operating room and among friends and colleagues. From "Four out of five urologists smell their apple juice before they drink it," to "What did the urologist say to the patient who forgot to take his medicine? Urine trouble!" Well, if you're reading this chapter, you just might have urine trouble. If that's the case, rest at ease. There are many reasons you might be having urine trouble, most are easily treated, and if you do have a serious disorder, you're living in the best medical era of all time and there are many treatment options for even the most serious cases.

One of the more common reasons a patient is referred to a urologist is because they have blood in their urine, a condition known as "hematuria." For the patient, blood in the urine is quite frightening, but blood in the urine doesn't necessarily mean there's a serious problem. But it is important to find out why there is blood in the urine.

Although the urologist usually has a good idea why the patient was referred and what the primary care provider's (PCP's) concerns were, we like to have a good understanding of what the patient has experienced. For that reason, I usually start my visit with a conversation that goes something like this.

"Hi, Mr. SoandSo, I'm Dr. Lieberman. How are you today and how can I help you?"

The patient will usually greet me politely, but their face will be serious. "I have blood in my urine, doc. I hope it's nothing serious."

Of course, they are usually pretty worried that it is indeed serious. My next question is aimed at learning more about just how serious it might be. In most cases, I'm able to alleviate their concerns, but they need to have it checked out. Blood in the urine isn't something to ignore.

"How do you know that you have blood in your urine?" I ask. The answer will give me important information.

It's at this point that the conversation will diverge in several potential directions, which is why it's important to ask the question. Hematuria presents in a variety of ways, and how it presents gives us clues to what is going on.

The responses might be, "I saw some a week ago, and then it went away. My urine is clear now, but I thought I should get it checked, just in case." Or, "I had burning and was peeing all the time, and then I saw some blood. They gave me antibiotics and it cleared up, but they referred me to you, it's probably just from my UTI, right?"

In some cases, they didn't know they had blood in their urine until their PCP told them. "My doctor did a UA," they might say, referring to a urine analysis, "and told me I have microscopic blood, but I've never seen it." Or maybe it's more along the lines of, "I've had microscopic blood in my urine for years and they've given me all kinds of tests, IVP's (kidney x-rays with IV contrast or dye), CT scans, cystoscopies (a procedure done in the office under local anesthesia in which a flexible 5mm scope is passed through the urethra to the bladder), but they never find anything. That's why I've come to you. I need to know what's wrong." And in some cases, the patient has come straight to me after peeing a stream of urine as red as cabernet wine. Whatever the case, it's my job to determine where that blood is coming from and why it's there in the first place.

It's not uncommon for me to have already taken a look at their urine before I've even met the patient. We normally obtain a urine specimen before the exam, and I would at times look at it prior to taking a history and doing a physical. It doesn't take much blood for urine to look pink, so with just one glance I can tell before it's even tested if there's blood. They taught us in medical school that if you couldn't read a newspaper through it (back in the days when newspapers were printed on paper, and not on computer screens!), then there was a significant amount of blood. Sometimes the specimen has clotted blood in it, which is an even greater concern. Whatever the state of the urine, if you can tell at a glance that the urine contains blood, it's called "gross hematuria."

Conversely, if the blood is not visible to the human eye and can only be observed through a microscope, we call it "microscopic hematuria." Whether you submit a urine specimen to the lab or we analyze it in the office, the specimen is first tested with a dipstick. The test strips measure not only blood, but also glucose, bilirubin, urobilinogen (two liver tests), ketones, leukocytes (white blood cells, which could indicate infection), nitrites (indicating the presence of bacteria), protein, and pH.

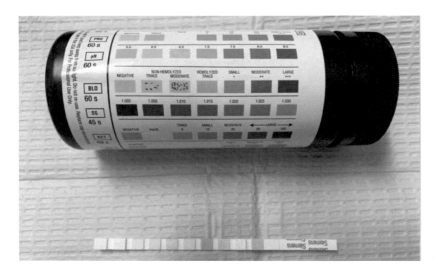

The first part of a UA (urine analysis) is the dipstick. When the "blo" box turns green, it indicates the presence of blood.

If the dipstick is positive for blood, the amount of blood is indicated by how dark green the dipstick box for blood becomes. The microscopic exam of the urine (done in most urologists' offices) will give us an accurate measure of the concentration of blood, or how many red blood cells are seen in each high-powered field. The specimen it then spun in a centrifuge, which concentrates the solid particles in the urine toward the bottom of the test tube. Those particles are put on a slide and either the lab tech or urologist (or both) examines it under a microscope, analyzing the number of red and white blood cells, crystals, and "casts" (think of a bunch of red or white cells stuck in a tube to form a "cast" of cells).

One thing that can complicate a UA (urine analysis) is how the urine specimen was obtained. Instructions are usually given to patients on how to collect the specimen, but sometimes the specimen is still contaminated by vaginal or external genitalia blood. We can usually tell when the specimen has been contaminated because there will be cells present that usually aren't present in urine. For most circumcised men this contamination is not as common as what's seen in women due to improper collection.

Hematuria is sometimes associated with other symptoms - pain with urination, urinary frequency, urgency, frequently getting up at night to pee (nocturia), or pain anywhere along the course of the urinary tract from the kidney to the tip of the urethra. Sometimes hematuria will not be associated with any symptoms. This is called asymptomatic hematuria. Hematuria can also be chronic or acute. Why is any of this classification important? Why does it matter? If you have blood in your urine, shouldn't you see a urologist and have some tests to figure out why?

It matters because you don't want to have tests and X-rays that aren't necessary. Conversely, there are situations when you want to know what's causing the blood in the urine because there are certain conditions, particularly bladder and kidney cancer, that can be cured if diagnosed early, and possibly not cured if the diagnosis is delayed. Depending on what type of hematuria a person has, will determine the work up. Let's consider each type of hematuria starting with asymptomatic microscopic hematuria.

Microscopic Hematuria

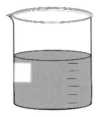

Gross hematuria means blood can be seen in the urine.

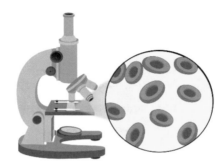

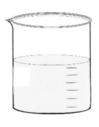

Microscopic hematuria means blood can be seen only with a microscope.

Gross and microscopic hematuria

Asymptomatic microhematuria means that not only is there no visible blood in the urine, but blood has been found in the lab tests your physician ordered. If you've had no symptoms and couldn't see the blood, chances are you've been surprised by the lab results and you're worried that some silent killer might be lurking inside somewhere. Fortunately, that is usually not the case.

When I was in training, we were taught that any sign of microhematuria, no matter how negligible, required a thoroug and often uncomfortable workup that required an IVP and rigid cystoscopy (and often retrograde pyelograms - see glossary). It turns out, however, that small amounts of blood in the urine is quite common. Depending on how presence of blood is defined, the prevalence of blood in the urine is between 9% and 18% of patients, and an estimated 25,000,000 Americans have blood in their urine. Blood in the urine is more common in older people and in smokers, but that doesn't mean there is anything wrong with them (although smoking is a definite risk factor for bladder cancer, which we discuss in Chapter 9).

In 2010, Ron Loo, M.D., one of my colleagues at Kaiser in southern California, and I found that in over one million urinalyses done at Kaiser Southern California, almost one-third had evidence of hematuria, yet the evidence of bladder cancer for this same sample was less than one percent! We concluded that doing a urinalysis as a screening test for bladder or kidney cancer was a waste of time and resources—and was especially a disservice to our patients, because many of them were subjected to radiation from CT scans, and uncomfortable cystoscopies.

"Perhaps," you might be thinking, "but if there's even a slight chance of cancer, shouldn't follow-up tests be a good thing?" Not necessarily. Just think about it. I had been evaluating tens of thousands (or more) patients with asymptomatic microscopic hematuria for more than 35 years and never finding anything. But because I'd been trained that any indication of hematuria required a series of follow-up tests, these patients who had no other signs or symptoms of a disorder, and only trace amounts of microscopic blood in their urine, were subjected to tests with potential harmful radiation and dyes injected into them. They all had cystoscopy, which could be uncomfortable (particularly rigid cystoscopes we used in the 70s and 80s), and they had to take time off from work. Depending on their insurance some often had to pay hundreds, maybe thousands of dollars in co-pays and deductibles. Some of them, like airline pilots, whose routine flight physicals may have turned up microscopic blood in the urine, were unable to return to work until we cleared them. Yet even though I could predict with 99% accuracy that they were perfectly fine, they were subjected to these unnecessary test, as well as all that worry.

For those who did have cancer, there were always other signs and symptoms. For those patients, additional tests made sense. But for those who just have microscopic traces of blood in their urine with no other symptoms? My opinion was that we were subjecting patients to unnecessary radiation and cystoscopy. Why then did we do it?

First, it was the standard of care at that time, and the one recommended by the American Urologic Association. Second, there was no financial incentive for either radiologists or urologists to rock the boat and say that a work-up for asymptomatic microhematuria was probably not necessary. Anyone who did rock that boat would be met with resistance from within the profession. Third, patients expected follow-up tests when blood was found and telling them they didn't need the tests, especially in light of the professional standards of the time would leave them feeling they were not getting adequate care. And finally, there was always the potential for litigation.

Some urologists would say (some still do say) that if they didn't evaluate a patient with asymptomatic microscopic hematuria and that patient was later diagnosed with cancer, then the physician who failed to the CT scan and cystoscopy could be on the hook for a malpractice suit. So we erred on the side of caution and maintained a standard of care that subjected many patients to costly, uncomfortable, and sometimes risky tests that rarely revealed any serious problem. For years I was concerned that these tests were unnecessary. My fellow Kaiser urology chiefs and I launched a national study involving all Kaiser regions to determine how many patients with asymptomatic micro-hematuria had a serious problem. Our findings were more remarkable than I'd anticipated.

In the first year of the study, we collected data on 10,000 patients who had been referred by their PCP to a Kaiser urologist for "micro-scopic hematuria." We recorded six variables for all of these pa-tients—age, sex, smoking history, amount of microscopic blood in the urine, presence of absence of symptoms, and whether or not the pa-tient had a history of seeing blood in the urine with the naked eye (gross hematuria). All patients had cystoscopy and were subjected to imaging, usually a CT scan. We found that patients who had a history of gross hematuria were at the highest risk of having a malignancy. We were able to assign a risk score based on the variables of history of gross hematuria, sex (males are at greater risk), age (the older you are, the greater the risk), and smoking history. According to risk, we were able to divide the initial group of 10,000 into three groups based on risk factors (low, medium, and high). If a person had a history of gross hematuria within the past six months of being seen, they could not be in the low risk group.

There were 4,400 patients in the low risk group and only three malignancies were found among them. I went back and personally re-viewed those three cases and it turns out that two of them did not have a malignancy after all, and one had a history of gross hematuria a year prior, but not in the past six months. Of the 10,000 in the initial group, 52 did have cancer, but all of them had a history of gross hematuria, and all were in the high risk group.

All this is to say, if your physician tells you that your lab work reveals blood in your urine and you've never noticed any indication of blood (that is, you've never had gross hematuria) and you have NO symptoms, it's highly unlikely that it's anything serious. On the other hand CT scans involve a lot of radiation, which can cause cancer, so why have a test that you don't need?

I presented our findings at the annual American Urological Association meeting in 2013, and after the presentation, I sat down next to a urologist from Great Britain. He leaned over and said, "Very interesting talk, but we don't work up microhematuria in Europe, zero, none." Whether that is because they've known for some time that the workup for asymptomatic microhematuria is unnecessary, or that we have a privatized medical system that profits from expensive tests, it's hard to say.

As a result of our study, we developed a guideline at Kaiser for evaluating microscopic hematuria that has significantly reduced the number of unnecessary CT scans, cystoscopies, and days off work for unnecessary tests and appointments with a urologist. As a result of these new guidelines, we alleviated a lot of needless worry, not to mention the discomfort and financial strain of needless tests. But suppose the microscopic urine isn't the only thing going on? What if you have symptoms? If that's the case, you may indeed want further tests.

Microscopic Blood in Urine with Other Symptoms

If you have microscopic blood in your urine along with other symptoms, we call it *symptomatic* microhematuria. What symptoms are we talking about? They can be specific to the urinary tract—pain or burning with urination, frequent urination, urgency, for example—or they may be more generalized "total body" symptoms such as fever, lethargy, malaise, or weakness. It's not uncommon for someone to go to their doctor for these generalized symptoms, have the doctor recommend a diagnostic workup, including blood and urine tests, and find the microscopic blood in the urine. In this case, a work-up is necessary.

Pain anywhere along the course of the urinary tract would trigger a urinary analysis (UA). This might be pain with the flank (kidneys, adrenals, ureters, and anything else in the retroperitoneum). Pain above the pubic bone could indicate a bladder infection. To learn more, it's important to consider your health history. Do you have a history of kidney stones? If so, there's a good chance that may explain the pain and hematuria. Maybe you have a history of UTI's? Whatever is going on, it's not something you can diagnose yourself, so you do need to see a doctor. Your physician will take history and order a urinary analysis. Based on what's found in that analysis if this is your first UTI, your doctor will treat your UTI and then recheck your urine for blood after the infection has resolve. If there is no UTI, a CT urogram will be done to see if the hematuria may be explained by kidney stones or something else. And, you will need to see a urologist for cystoscopy in order to diagnosis the cause of your symptomatic microhematuria.

Other symptoms might include frequent urination, burning with urination, urgency (feeling like you gotta go right now!), and getting up frequently at night to pee. These symptoms, when associated with microhematuria, might indicate bladder cancer, and should be evaluated with a CT scan and cystoscopy. Symptomatic hematuria can also be associated with Benign Prostatic Hyperplasia (BPH), which is an enlarged prostate that may be constricting the urethra. Chapter 5 is the chapter on BPH.

Whether or not you have other symptoms, what if the blood wasn't microscopic? If you notice blood in your urine, there still may not be a serious problem, but you definitely want to find out what's wrong.

Visible Blood in the Urine – Gross Hematuria

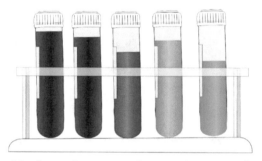

Various degrees of gross hematuria

If you do see blood in your urine, you need to see a urologist. This condition is called gross hematuria. The blood may include visible clots, or can look like coffee grounds or cola. It may be pale pink, bright cherry red, dark burgundy, or bright orange. If the blood in your urine looks like coffee grounds, it's "old blood," meaning you are not actively bleeding, and the blood is likely coming from either the kidneys, bladder, or prostate. If the blood in your urine is bright red, however, it means you are actively bleeding. Sometimes, particularly with bladder cancers, the blood clots can be so voluminous that they will completely obstruct the bladder outlet and the patient can't pee at all. This is called clot retention and requires a urologist to irrigate the clots out, which requires a trip to the ER or urologists office. In my experience that this is no fun for either the patient or the urologist.

Gross hematuria can occur at the beginning, middle, or end of the stream, or be present throughout the stream. If you notice blood in your urine, try to note when it happens, because that bit of history can be helpful in trying to determine where the blood is coming from. If the bleeding is at the beginning of the stream and then clears, it's usually anywhere from the prostate or prostatic urethra, along the course of the urethra to the tip of the penis. If the blood is originated in the urethra, it will sometimes show up in the underwear.

This is true for women, as well, but the story is a little different for them. Women sit down to pee and then see the blood in the toilet. If they aren't menstruating, they may assume that the blood is in the urine, but it may have come from the uterus, cervix, or vagina. Women are also more prone to urinary tract infections, which can be associated with gross hematuria.

If the blood appears in a steady stream, or begins clear and turns dark, then the problem could be further up in your genitourinary tract. Your urologist will want to check your kidneys and bladder with a CT and cystoscopy. While there is certainly cause for concern, the problem could be from an infection or stone, but it could also be something more serious like kidney or bladder cancer.

As you can see, blood in the urine takes many forms. To keep it simple, if you are told "you have blood in your urine" you might be initially alarmed, but if you have no symptoms and have never seen blood in your urine, rest assured that you likely have nothing significantly wrong. However, if you *do* see blood in your urine, please seek professional medical help soon. If you have symptoms and your doctor says you have microscopic blood in your urine and recommends further evaluation, I'd advise that you do it, whether it's a renal ultrasound or CT urogram, and a visit to the urologist for a 15 minute procedure called cystoscopy.

A CT urogram is a CT scan that makes it possible to visualize the kidneys, ureters and bladder. For the procedure, a dye will be injected into your arm or hand, so that the radiologist can observe how it courses through and lights up the kidneys, then drains down the ureters and into the bladder. You may feel a rush of warmth from the dye but the procedure itself is painless, aside from the prick of the needle at the injection site.

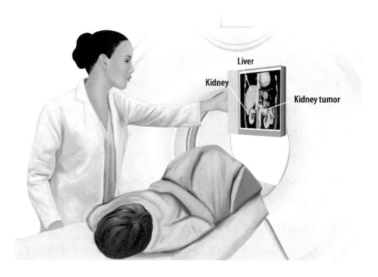

CT scan of kidneys showing right kidney tumor and thrombus (clot) in renal vein

Cystoscopy involves your urologist inserting a flexible 5 mm fiber optic scope into your urethra and up to your bladder. You'll be asked to empty your bladder. Your genitals will be prepped with a sterilizing solution (usually iodine based). A local anesthetic gel will be instilled into your urethra and held in place with a special clamp (in men). You won't see the urologist for 10-15 minutes while the numbing agent does it's thing. Once your urethra is numb, the urologist will insert the scope, which is attached to a camera. An image (your urethra and bladder) is displayed on a screen, so you both can see what's up there. Then sterile water will flow through the scope into your bladder and fill your bladder to give your urologist a good view. You'll feel like you have to pee, but try to relax and hold it. I know the procedure sounds awful, but you'll have to trust me on this one, it's not that bad. I've had four cystoscopies for gross blood in my urine due to stones in my prostate. It's mildly uncomfortable but not particularly painful.

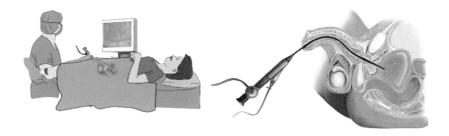

Flexible Cystoscopy in Men

Conclusion

While you absolutely need to see a doctor whenever you see blood in your urine, don't panic. The cause could well be from something benign. Blood in the urine means something is going on with the genitourinary tract, but that something might be a urinary tract infection (UTI), kidney or bladder stones (excruciating, but temporary), an enlarged prostate, a sexually transmitted disease (STD's), and can even be caused by some medications (blood thinners, sulfa containing drugs, etc). In other words, there might be a serious problem, but chances are, it's not. Nonetheless, don't wait—the sooner you know why you have blood in your urine, the sooner you can get started on an early course of treatment if it is serious. In subsequent chapters I'll discuss these more serious concerns should it turn out that you have a tumor one of your kidneys, bladder, prostate or elsewhere in your genitourinary tract. But for now, know that microscopic blood in the urine is common, and in most cases, not an indication of cancer, especially if there are no symptoms associated with it. If you can see it, it is a literal red flag giving you a shot at early detection.

But what if your problem isn't blood in your urine at all. What if your problem is you can't pee at all? If that's the problem, you have a blockage and we can help. In Chapter 5, I'll discuss some possible causes of urinary tract blockages, and possible fixes. For now, in the next chapter, let's take a closer look at urinary tract infections.

CHAPTER 4

Urinary Tract Infections

An infection caused by a bug. That bug can be a bacteria, a virus, fungus, or other rare germs. Infections cause the body to mount an inflammatory response in an attempt to rid the body of the bug. However, you can have inflammation without an infection, that is, sometimes we can't identify an organism or bug that's producing the inflammation.

A urologist will be able to tell the difference by doing urine analyses and cultures. How can you tell whether your urinary problem rises to the level of seeing a doctor or urologist? As we discussed in the last chapter, anytime you see blood in your urine, you need to see a urologist. Similarly, anytime you have pain when you pee, you need to see a doctor. But first, let's take a closer look at urinary tract infections (UTI), so that you have a better idea of why we want you to seek treatment as soon as possible.

Men don't get many urinary infections without good reason, particularly men under the age of 50. If you do get one, it's never fun. The infection can be anywhere along the genitourinary tract, including the kidneys, bladder, prostate, ureters, urethra, and organs within the scrotum (testicles and epididymis). An infection in the bladder or urethra is considered a lower tract infection, while an infection in kidneys or prostate is an upper tract infection. Lower tract infections are caused by bacteria that enter the urethra then migrate into the bladder. Though rare in men (only about three percent of men will ever have a UTI in their lifetime), when they do occur, they can become complicated and often reach the kidneys or bladder, so they're nothing to mess around with. Though most cases UTI's can initially be treated with antibiotics, and can be perfectly well managed and resolved by a primary care provider (PCP), there's a reason or cause for a UTI in a man, so my opinion is that all men with a documented bacterial UTI should see a urologist.

These symptoms of a UTI are unpleasant at best and can include abdominal pain, burning when urinating, fever, cloudy or bloody urine, increased urgency, urgency without being able to pee, and smelly urine. Serious UTIs in men can be associated with fever, chills, nausea, vomiting, or back pain. If you have these symptoms and are diagnosed with a UTI, you will need imaging (ultrasound of kidneys and bladder, or CT urogram) and a visit to a urologist.

One of the first steps your doctor will take is to determine what type of infection you have. There are many different kinds of UTIs, ranging from simple bladder infections to serious kidney infections or a kidney abscess. Some UTIs can become quite serious if the bacteria enter the bloodstream, in which case a condition called sepsis, or septic shock, can result, which is potentially deadly. For this reason, early diagnosis and treatment is imperative.

To assess the infection, your doctor may use a urine dipstick, discussed in the previous chapter, and/or have you provide a midstream urine sample to send to the lab. A midstream sample means that you begin peeing to clear the urethra, then the sample is taken from your midstream urine. Your doctor will also want to examine your genitals as well as palpate your abdominal area to feel for any lumps or tenderness. If your doctor does not do a rectal exam to feel your prostate when you are acutely ill, that's probably okay, because if the source of the infection is the prostate, pushing on it may push the bacteria into your bloodstream and cause sepsis.

If your infection is limited to the lower tract, it is often easily treated, but you want to catch it early so that it does not spread to the kidneys or bladder, where treatment can become more difficult.

We'll start by outlining the different types of urinary tract infections. Like I said above, it is always appropriate for a man with a UTI to be referred to a urologist, even after successful treatment by his PCP. Though women frequently get UTI's given their short urethras, when a man gets a UTI from something other than a sexually transmitted disease (STD - which can cause an infection in the urethra) there's usually a cause that needs to be addressed, such as stagnant urine in the bladder, a kidney or bladder stone, or a foreign body such as a broken off piece of catheter. There are other co-morbidities that contribute to UTIs in men (including neurologic conditions that predispose to stagnant urine, Crohn's disease and diabetes). If you have a UTI, you'll want to see a urologist to find out why.

Men who do get UTIs are at risk for developing recurrent UTIs, due to the underlying cause (such as having a disease or disorder predisposing to the infections). If you do develop recurring or chronic

UTIs, you will want to get evaluated anytime you are experiencing new symptoms.

Cystitis

When bacteria get into the bladder they set up camp and cause an immune response. We call that cystitis, commonly referred to as a bladder infection. The bacteria gain access to the bladder through the urethra, and can be caused by a number of factors - catheters, sexually transmitted diseases, difficulty emptying the bladder (stagnant urine), diabetes, and poor hygeine. Urinary tract infections can also be caused by a blockage in the urethra from a scar (urethral stricture), or from a foreign body like a catheter. Anytime there is stagnant urine in a man's bladder the urine serves as a breeding ground for bacteria.

When ascending bacteria get into the urethra they can cause an infection in the urethra or urethritis. Most of these infections are from sexually transmitted diseases and are due to chalmydia or gonococcal bacteria (gonnorhea), or a bug called *ureaplasma ureolyticum*. Other rare bugs can also cause urinary infections in men who have compromised immune systems. Most urethral infections are caused by STDs and can be treated by PCPs with antibiotics, and don't require the services of a urologist, unless they recur. Most urethral STD infections are treated by primary care providers with antibiotics, and don't require the services of a urologist, unless they recur. STD infections are usually uncomplicated, unlike infections that occur in the bladder or kidney in men, which are a more serious concern and will need to be further evaluated by a urologist.

If you picked up a UTI from a sexually transmitted disease, the symptoms are typically limited to pain in the urethra and a discharge. One of the late complications that occurs after an infection in the urethra is that scar tissue, called a urethral stricture, can develop after urethritis. The narrowing in the urethra can be quite significant and appear like a pinpoint opening, whereas normally the inner diameter of the urethra is equivalent to a straw. A stricture that occurs after a bout of urethritis will usually result in one or more urinary symptoms: a slow trickling stream, difficulty starting a stream, frequent urination, getting the urge to go an feeling like you can't hold it, or feeling like you can't empty your bladder.

Cystitis in a male is usually associated with some other problem that has caused or contributed to the infection, which is why any man with cystitis should see a urologist. Some examples include an enlarged prostate (see Chapter 5), which can occasionally prevent the bladder from emptying completely resulting in stagnant urine, making it possible for bacteria to grow and set up shop.

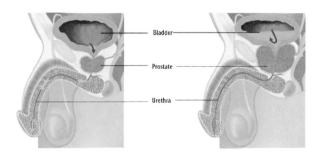

Male Lower Urinary Tract – (L) normal, (R) benign prostate enlargement with obstruction of prostatic urethra

Another cause of cystitis is an anatomic anomaly called a bladder diverticulum. This diverticulum can either be hereditary, or develop, and is a small, or not so small, sac or pouch in the bladder where urine pools and doesn't empty, again, allowing bacteria to grow. I've seen bladder diverticula that are twice the size of the actual bladder and hold up to a liter of stagnant urine—it's not hard to imagine how the bacteria that can take up residence in such a situation.

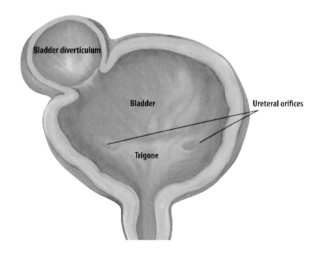

Bladder Diverticulum

Finally, yet another cause of cystitis is a bladder stone(s). Bladder stones can be solitary or multiple and can range in size from a BB to as large as a tennis ball.— INSERT FIG 46 — Infections can also be caused by foreign bodies in the bladder. Usually these are pieces of previously-placed urinary catheters or stents that have broken off and have not passed. Another possibility, if you have had a surgical procedure for an enlarged prostate (such as the TURP, discussed in the following chapter), is that pieces of tissue from the prostate have remained in the bladder. Finally, an infection of the prostate, which lies just below the bladder, can easily reach the bladder and infect it. If the prostate is infected, you have a condition known as prostatitis.

Prostatitis

One of our concerns when patients come to us with a UTI is that the infection has spread from the prostate to the bladder or kidneys. When the infection starts in the prostate, you may develop prostatitis, which is another type of UTI that occurs in men characterized by symptoms similar to cystitis: frequent urination, urgency, sometimes burning, nocturia (frequent peeing at night), and pain above the pubic bone and/or in the perineum (the space between the scrotum and prostate). There can also be pain in the penis, abdomen, scrotum and genitalia and even flu-like symptoms. Only 10% of prostate infections are from bacteria. Prostatitis caused by bacteria is frequently associated with cystitis (bacterial bladder infection) and symptoms are similar to those seen with cystitis—grossly cloudy urine, occasionally visual blood in the urine. A severe infection can progress to an abscess of the prostate or spread to the bloodstream and cause sepsis and septic shock. It you do have acute prostatitis, it's a good idea for your doctor to refrain from doing a rectal exam until the infection has been adequately treated. Most men with documented acute bacterial prostatitis will want to see a urologist.

If bacterial prostatitis makes up only 10% of all cases of prostatitis, what about the other 90%? There are three other categories of prostatitis—chronic bacterial, chronic non-bacterial, and prostatodynia. Inflammation of the prostate is what defines prostatitis. If you have symptoms of inflammation of the prostate, but a normal UA, and you are not responding to antibiotic treatment by your PCP, you may want to be referred to a urologist for evaluation, diagnosis, and treatment. It may be that you have chronic bacterial prostatitis, and will respond to a different or more intensive antibiotic treatment. But, if there are no bacteria to account for the symptoms and inflammation, then you'll want to avoid antibiotics so that you don't develop antibiotic resistance.

So how does your urologist know which you have? When testing your urine, the first 10-20 ccs of urine will reveal what is going on in your urethra. If your urine from your urethra is infected, you likely have urethritis. Your midstream urine will indicate what is going on in your bladder and kidneys. If that urine is infected, you either have cystitis or a kidney infection (pyelonephritis). If your urologist does a prostate massage to obtain secretions from your prostate (something that should *never* be done if acute bacterial prostatitis is suspected), and upon a microscopic examination finds white blood cells present, you have an inflammation in your prostate—in other words, you have chronic prostatitis. If the secretions contain bacteria, then you are likely suffering from chronic *bacterial* prostatitis and will require a three to six week course of antibiotics. On the other hand, if your urologist notes inflammation but no infection, then you likely have chronic nonbacterial prostatitis.

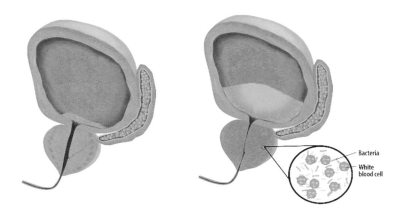

Bacteria

White
blood cell

Normal Prostate (L), Bacterial Prostatitis, chronic or acute (R)

It sometimes turns out that even though there is pain in the prostate, there are no inflammatory cells, no signs of infection or bacteria. If that is the case, the diagnosis is prostatodynia, a frustrating diagnosis for both patient and urologist, because it requires additional testing to find out what's going on. These tests can include examining the urethra, prostate and bladder with a cystoscope, or even an MRI, to make sure there's nothing more serious going on. Among the more serious concerns is an infection of the kidneys.

Pyelonephritis

A bacterial infection can reach the kidney or kidneys one of two ways, either by ascending from the bladder to the kidney through the ureter (the tube that connects the kidney to the bladder), or via the bloodstream. A kidney infection is called pyelonephritis. Pyelonephritis can be serious. It is characterized by flank pain (pain in the kidney), and sometimes fever, nausea, and vomiting. So how does a man get a kidney infection? It gets back to the three possible causes of all UTIs in men—stagnant urine, stones, or foreign bodies.

A kidney infection in a man can also be associated with obstruction of the ureter anywhere along the one foot length of ureter from kidney to bladder, which in turn causes stagnant urine. The obstruction can be due to a stone, an acquired or congenital abnormality, or what we call an extrinsic cause. That means there is something outside the urinary tract that is causing the blockage. There are a variety of things that can cause this ranging from benign enlargement of lymph nodes, to scaring from prior radiation therapy of the pelvis, to cancer. Other causes can include an infection from elsewhere in the body entering the bloodstream and reaching the kidneys.

Pyelonephritis needn't be serious, if caught early. It can usually be treated with a course of antibiotics and clear up in one to two weeks, *provided the cause of the infection has been addressed.* If not diagnosed and treated early, however, the infection can cause permanent damage to your kidneys and develop into an abscess. What's more, if the bacteria enter your bloodstream, you may develop sepsis which, as I've stated earlier, can cause shock and even be fatal. Because infections can cause scarring to the kidneys, if left untreated or if the treatment is delayed or incomplete, the infection could lead to high blood pressure, chronic kidney disease and renal failure.

Pyelonephritis can also be caused by stones in one of two ways. Stones made of magnesium, ammonium, and phosphate make up what is called "infectious or struvite stone," that has a specific bacteria in it (*e. coli, pseudomonas,* or *proteus*). The only way to clear up the infection is to get rid of the stone. The other cause of pyelonephritis is an obstruction of urine drainage or a blockage anywhere along the drainage system from the junction of the renal pelvis and ureter, to the end of the penile urethra. When a blockage of urine drainage results in stagnant urine, an infection can occur. Finally, just as in the bladder, diverticula can also occur in the kidney and become infected.

Because UTIs in men are likely to have an underlying cause, men who don't see a urologist tend to get recurring infections, which are then treated with different antibiotics, leading to antibiotic resistance, so it's important to see a urologist even after your first UTI.

Bacteriuria

It's also possible to have bacteria in the urine and not have a UTI. This condition is called bacteriuria. Bacteria are in the bladder and urine but do not cause an infection or inflammation. Instead, they are passed into the toilet with urination or by emptying the bladder through a catheter. The condition of bacteriuria without a flagrant UTI is seen in some men with chronic indwelling catheters or double J stents. The urine is colonized by bacteria but you may not have any symptoms. If this is the case, it's not be a good idea to treat the bacteria with antibiotics, because treating bacterial colonization when it's not causing any harm leads to bacterial resistance to antibiotics. This is a huge problem not only in the area of UTIs but conditions such as upper respiratory infections (bronchitis, pneumonia, sinus infections, etc) where symptoms are caused by viruses, not bacteria, yet antibiotics are given.

Epididymitis

One final concern with UTIs is an infection of the epididymis. I refer you back to chapter one on anatomy. The epididymis is a caterpillar-sized structure that sits behind the testicle and transports sperm from the testicle to the epididymis. The epididymis is attached to the prostate by the vas deferens. Pathogens (such as bacteria or viruses) can invade the epididymis by traveling from the bladder, prostate, or urethra down the vas, or or get into the vas via the bloodstream, causing an infection known as epididymitis.

Acute epididymitis usually occurs in men between the ages of 15 and 40 and is diagnosed 600,000 times in the United States each year. It is considered a sexually transmitted disease if it's caused by gonorrhea or chlamydia, sexually transmitted organisms and common culprits. Sexual partners can give the bugs to one another, so they should also be informed and treated.

Any urinary tract infection organism can cause epididymitis. If a bug is identified, the most appropriate antibiotic will be prescribed. If no bug is identified, then the choice of antibiotic is based on what would be the most likely organism. The most common bacteria that cause epididymitis are sensitive to doxycycline, ciprofloxacin, and trimethoprim/sulfa, so your physician is likely to prescribe one of those.

Other local measures can help the pain, including elevating the scrotum on some towels, ice packs (bags of frozen peas work great), non-steroidal anti-inflammatory medication (Advil, Motrin), Tylenol, and the standard medical advice for any ailment to "drink lots of fluids."

If you think you might have epididymitis, you want to get it treated, because delayed treatment, or no treatment can lead to an abscess or "pus pocket" that may require surgical drainage, or even necessitate removal of the epididymis and/or testes. It's not common, but delayed treatment can also cause infertility.

Treatment is usually 10-14 days, though you should start feeling better in 3 to 5 days. (Remember, even if the symptoms have disappeared, the bacteria have not, so you must take the full course of antibiotics.) The pain should improve but can sometimes last for weeks to even months. And you should consult with your doctor as far as resuming sexual activity and whether or not your partner needs to be treated.

Although a UTI or STD can cause epididymitis, epididymitis does not necessarily mean you have been infected with a bug. If there is an obstruction or blockage between the epididymis and urethra, the back pressure from the obstruction can result in significant inflammation, swelling, and pain in the epididymis. The most common cause of such an obstruction is vasectomy, and this complication occurs in 1 -3 % of men undergoing a vasectomy. It's unclear whether there is an infectious component to the problem, so treatment with antibiotics is at the discretion of the urologist. Other obstructive processes at the level of the prostate or urethra can also be a cause.

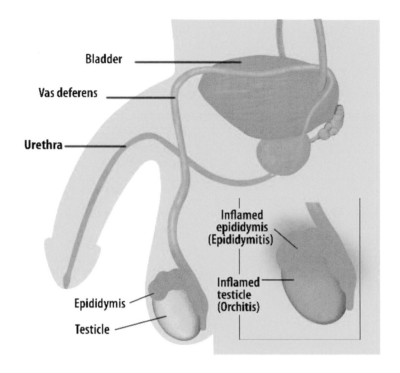

Bladder

Vas deferens

Urethra

Inflamed
epididymis
(Epididymitis)

Inflamed
testicle
(Orchitis)

Epididymis

Testicle

Epididymitis, chronic or acute

Mumps is a well know viral cause of epididymal orchitis. The vaccine for mumps was introduced in 1967, and then combined with a vaccine for measles and rubella (German measles) in 1971 (the MMR vaccine). In 1995 the varicella (chicken pox) vaccine was added (the MMRV vaccine). I was born in 1951, before the vaccine, and I distinctly remember having chicken pox when I was 5 or 6, and then measles when I was 8. I remember being pretty ill with measles for about a week and missing a St Louis Cardinal double header with the Cincinnati Reds (the Cardinals won the double header, Bob Gibson pitched in one of the games). I escaped mumps, but I knew several friends who didn't. None of them talked about scrotal swelling or pain, but I guess pre-adolescent and adolescent boys aren't prone to sharing such information.

Despite how common mumps once were, I didn't know that mumps caused epididymitis until medical school. Thanks to MMR and now MMRV vaccines, mumps is now rare. However, with all the misinformation around COVID vaccines, I'm afraid there may be more anti-vax sentiment toward the MMRV vaccines, which up until now have saved countless lives and have prevented even more morbidity.

What morbidity? Well, boys who get mumps have a 1 in 3 chance of having epididymitis. The resulting inflammation can result in shrinking or atrophy of the testicle, to the degree that it turns into the size of a pea. That testicle will no longer make testosterone or sperm. In addition, a common response seen in post-pubescent boys is their bodies form antibodies that attack not just the virus but also testicular tissue. This immune response results in infertility a few years later. In my practice, I've seen plenty of men my age who had mumps during childhood or adolescence with tiny testicles due to mumps.

Acute epididymitis can become chronic epididymitis. The bugs have been eliminated but the inflammation and pain persist for three months or more. Treatment is non-steroidal anti-inflammatory medication for a month. If this fails, sometimes surgical removal of the epididymis is considered. All this is to say, having a UTI can lead to more serious issues, as well as have a more serious cause, so if you develop a UTI, don't mess around. Get a proper diagnosis and treatment.

Conclusion

In closing, if you are a man with a UTI, your PCP will treat you with an appropriate antibiotic. Because most UTIs in men are due to stagnant urine from an obstruction anywhere in the urinary tract, or stone (both infectious or non-infectious), or a foreign body, it's still *important that you see a urologist*. Expect that prior to your appointment, an imaging study (usually a CT urogram) will be done. When you do see a urologist, s/he will do whatever tests are necessary to figure out why you got a UTI in the first place. These tests will likely include an ultrasound of your bladder to see how much urine is left in your bladder after you pee, and cystoscopy to have a look at your urethra, the inside part of your prostate (the prostatic urethra), and the bladder.

In men over 50, UTI's are often caused by a blockage that results in stagnant urine. The blockage can often come from an enlarged prostate, also known as BPH, which is usually a benign and treatable but discomforting blockage. In the next chapter, we turn to a closer look at BPH or Benign Prostate Hyperplasia, what it means if you have it, and your treatment options.Rest assured that whatever the cause, we can find out and fix it.

CHAPTER 5

Can't Pee? See Me

Imagine you're at a ballgame. It's a beautiful day and you're enjoying a beer as you watch the Seattle Mariners and the Texas Rangers square off. You've been looking forward to this game all week, but now that you're in the bleachers, you can hardly stay awake. You didn't sleep well because you kept having to get up to pee. Even now it hasn't stopped. It's the top of the 6th and you've already been to the bathroom three times since the game began, but you don't think you can hold it a second longer.

"Gotta go, be right back," you tell your family as you hustle to the bathroom, afraid you won't make it in time and you'll wet your pants. Yet once you're standing there with your pants unzipped, nothing happens. The intense urge to pee is still there, powerful as ever, but all that comes out is a weak dribble that starts and stops. You finally feel like you're finished and head back, but by then there are two outs in the top of the sixth and the Mariners have taken the lead on a two-run homer that you missed. The inning finishes and the Rangers come to bat in the bottom of the sixth, but you can't stay to watch. You have to pee again.

If this story sounds like something that might be happening to you, you're not alone. As men age into their sixties and seventies, most will have some form of difficulty urinating. The symptoms usually come on slowly and gradually as we age, and at first may not be too concerning. You might find that rather than feeling like the gush of a firehose, you pee with a slow, thin stream. You might get up once in the night, nearly every night, but that's all. Or it might be like the example above, where you get little sleep, and dare not wander too far from a toilet because you know you'll need one sooner, rather than later. If that's the case, your quality of life is affected day and night.

If you have these symptoms, you may have an enlarged prostate. The clinical diagnosis for an enlarged prostate gland is benign prostatic hyperplasia (BPH), which is is a pathologic diagnosis that denotes a swelling of the prostate. Of course, these symptoms don't always mean that your prostate is enlarged. It could be inflamed or infected—a condition known as prostatitis that may require antibiotics. Your urinary troubles could also be a side effect from a medication, antihistamines for example. The first thing you want to do is determine if your symptoms are medically significant and you need to see a doctor.

Depending on the severity of your symptoms, how bothered you are by them, and whether or not the problem adversely affects your bladder and kidney function, it's a problem that can often be treated and cured. This chapter will address whether or not you need to see a urologist, or if your primary care doctor can diagnose and then treat you. We'll discuss the types of medications used, and the wide variety of both minimally invasive and surgical treatments available.

If you're having trouble peeing, how do you know how serious it is? Should you see your primary care doctor, or go straight to a urologist? Is it dangerous to wait and see if it clears up on its own? There are subjective and objective criteria for assessing how bad things are, and there are ways of telling whether or not your symptoms are from an enlarged prostate or something else that may or may not be more serious. Let's consider how we assess your symptoms before taking action.

Subjectively, ask yourself how much are your symptoms bothering you. The following questionnaires can help assess your subjective experienceii. If you're have problems peeing, these questionnaires may help decide your next steps.

Global Question 1

Overall, how bothersome has any trouble with urination been during the last month?

0 – Not at all bothersome
1 – Bothers me a little
2 – Bothers me some
3 – Bothers me a lot

Global Question 2

If you were to spend the rest of your life with your prostate symptoms just as they are now, how would you feel about that?

0 – Delighted
1 – Pleased
2 – Mostly satisfied
3 – Mixed (about equally satisfied
    and dissatisfied)
4 – Mostly dissatisfied
5 – Unhappy
6 – Terrible

Calculator: International Prostatism Symptom Score (IPSS)

Over the past month, how often have you had a sensation of not emptying your bladder completely after you finished urinating?	
	Not at all (0 points)
	Less than 1 time in 5 (1 point)
	Less than half the time (2 points)
	About half the time (3 points)
	More than half the time (4 points)
	Almost always (5 points)
Over the past month, how often have you had to urinate again less than 2 hours after you finished urinating?	
	Not at all (0 points)
	Less than 1 time in 5 (1 point)
	Less than half the time (2 points)
	About half the time (3 points)
	More than half the time (4 points)
	Almost always (5 points)
Over the past month, how often have you found you stopped and started again several times when you urinated?	

	Not at all (0 points)
	Less than 1 time in 5 (1 point)
	Less than half the time (2 points)
	About half the time (3 points)
	More than half the time (4 points)
	Almost always (5 points)
Over the past month, how often have you found it difficult to postpone urination?	
	Not at all (0 points)
	Less than 1 time in 5 (1 point)
	Less than half the time (2 points)
	About half the time (3 points)
	More than half the time (4 points)
	Almost always (5 points)
Over the past month, how often have you had a weak urinary stream?	
	Not at all (0 points)
	Less than 1 time in 5 (1 point)
	Less than half the time (2 points)
	About half the time (3 points)
	More than half the time (4 points)

	Almost always (5 points)
Over the past month, how often have you had to push or strain to begin urination?	
	Not at all (0 points)
	Less than 1 time in 5 (1 point)
	Less than half the time (2 points)
	About half the time (3 points)
	More than half the time (4 points)
	Almost always (5 points)
Over the past month, how many times did you most typically get up to urinate from the time you went to bed at night until the time you got up in the morning?	
	None (0 points)
	1 time (1 point)
	2 times (2 points)
	3 times (3 points)
	4 times (4 points)
	5 or more times (5 points)

IPSS: Score

0 to 7 points:	Mild symptoms
8 to 19 points:	Moderate symptoms
20 to 35 points:	Severe symptoms

Tally up your scores on the above questionnaires. A general rule of thumb is if your bother score is 5 or more, and if your IPSS score is more than 7, it would be a good idea discuss your symptoms with your doctor. What's probably happening is that your prostate is enlarged, and there's a good chance you have BPH.

As a prostate enlarges it restricts and slows your urine flow. If that happens, your bladder has to work harder to empty. As with any muscle that gets bigger the more you use it, as the bladder muscle generates more pressure, it increases in size, or thickens. The thicker the walls of the bladder become, the less urine it can hold. And, if something is blocking your urinary tract, your bladder will not empty completely. By seeing how much your bladder holds and how much urine is left in your bladder after you've peed, your doctor will have an objective starting point to assess how your condition progresses. Checking to see how much urine is left in your bladder with a bladder scanner (ultrasound) is one objective measure of how serious the problem may be.

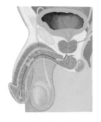
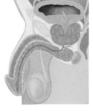
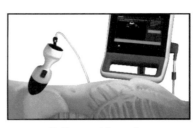

Normal prostate   BPH   Bladder scanner (ultrasound)

Bladder Ultrasound "Bladder Scanner" used to check post-void residual urine volume

Normally the prostate enlarges as men age, starting at age 50. BPH is rarely life threatening, and may not cause other medical problems. But, our guy at the game is really bothered by his BPH symptoms and the symptoms are adversely affecting his lifestyle. Plus, the longer he waits to do anything about his symptoms, the bigger he risks doing damage to his bladder and possibly kidneys. He needs to see a doctor—and so do you, if your symptoms are affecting your daily life activities and/or keeping you from getting enough rest at night. The first step is to make an appointment with your PCP.

Once you see your primary care physician, s/he will order some lab tests to include a urine analysis, PSA (Prostate Specific Antigen, which I'll tell you all about in Chapter 6), and kidney function tests (BUN and Creatinine), as well as other standard blood tests to rule out conditions like diabetes, problems with your electrolytes (sodium, potassium, chloride), and possibly other tests included in the panel (calcium, uric acid, phosphorus, a complete blood count, and liver function tests). Your physician may also discuss possible medications that can help with your symptoms.

Before sending you to see a urologist, your doctor may feel you simply need some symptomatic relief and prefer treating your symptoms with medication before any further tests are done. In many cases, however, s/he may want to order a simple ultrasound of your kidneys and what's called a post-void bladder (in other words, what's left in your bladder after you've peed like I mentioned above). The reason for an ultrasound is to look at your kidneys, particularly if there are any problems with the blood tests for kidney function. Your doctor wants to make sure that the inner part of each kidney, the collecting system (see Chapter 1 on Human Plumbing) isn't distended (enlarged) or dilated as a result of increased bladder pressure being transferred to the kidneys as the bladder tries to force urine through a blockage.

Now let's return to our guy at the ballgame. He has LUTS——Lower Urinary Tract Symptoms. His symptoms included frequent urination, hesitancy, trouble starting a stream, a slow, thin stop and start stream, and nocturia (getting up at night to pee). He is suffering from BOO—Bladder Outlet Obstruction. BOO is caused by anything that blocks urine from leaving the bladder, including an enlarged prostate. Other problem like a narrowing or restricting scar in the urethra (urethral stricture) can also cause symptoms of BOO. And if this alphabet soup is not confusing enough, there's BPO—Benign Prostatic Obstruction, BPE, Benign Prostatic Enlargement, and OAB, an Overactive Bladder.

There are two types of medications used to treat LUTS or BOO caused by BPH. These medications are sometimes used separately, and they are sometimes given together. If they work, and if your PSA shows that your risk of clinically significant prostate cancer is low (see

Chapter 6) then you probably don't need to see a urologist. If, however, your doctor is concerned that the condition is more serious, or if after examining your prostate, s/he is worried about how large it is, or if you don't respond to drugs, then you probably *should* see a urologist.

There are several reasons why you might choose to see urologist. The first is that you want to be sure that your symptoms are from typical benign prostate enlargement and not from something else like (prostate cancer, urethral stricture, neurologic problem causing bladder dysfunction, or other causes). These "other causes" can be potentially dangerous, but at the same time, they are often treatable. For example, a urethral stricture, which is a narrowing of the urethra (typically caused by catheters, STD's or injury to the scrotum or perineum), can have BOO the symptoms we see from BPH . Treatment of a urethral stricture is usually simple, quick, and effective, but if left untreated, a urethral stricture can cause irreparable bladder damage and even kidney failure. Another example would be prostate cancer. Early prostate cancer typically does not cause problems urinating, but because prostate cancer and BPH frequently coexist, early diagnosis and treatment is successful in producing a cure over 95% of the time (discussed in more detail in Chapter 6). Once you do see a urologist, what can you expect?

What to Expect When You See Your Urologist

When you first get to the urologist's office, if you haven't had a bladder ultrasound, you will. To do this test, usually performed in your urologist's office, you'll provide a urine sample, doing your best to completely empty your bladder. After you've done so, a nurse will come in with a small device like a microphone, put some lube above your pubic bone, then scan your bladder to get a volume measurement of how much urine remains in your bladder (what we call a post-void residual or PVR). The test takes less than a minute and is not painful or invasive in the least. The exam is an important objective measurement to determine how serious the BOO (bladder outlet obstruction) is.

Another objective measurement of how bad things are is a flow rate, which is how fast you urinate or how long it takes to empty your bladder. If the urologist wants this measurement, when you are asked to give the urine specimen, you'll pee into what is called a "flow meter." This meter registers the peak flow, and the average flow rate, and the volume you were able to empty, which is measured by how much is in the collection container. Once this is done, you'll have your bladder scanned.

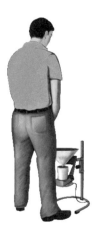

UroFlow Meter
measures peak and average urine flow in milliliters/sec

Unless there are no other reasons, (say you saw blood in your urine), at this point you usually would not need cystoscopy (a look in the bladder with a flexible scope and camera).

Based on your subjective symptoms (your bother score and IPSS from the charts above) and the objective data (ultrasound post-void residual, flow rate, rectal exam, PSA, BUN, creatinine levels), your urologist may talk to you about options. Those options include medications, non-invasive procedures, or invasive procedures. Let's take a closer look at each.

Medications

If you do have BOO due to BPH, there are two types of medications that may help: alpha blockers and 5 alpha reductase inhibitors. Flomax is the alpha blocker I commonly used, but there are others. The most commonly prescribed alpha blockers are:

- Alfuzosin (Uroxatral)
- Doxazosin (Cardura)
- Prazosin (Minipress)
- Silodosin (Rapaflo)
- Tamsulosin (Flomax)
- Terazosin (Hytrin)

Generally speaking, for moderate symptoms most patients are started on alpha blockers first. Alpha blockers work by blocking the neurotransmitter which causes smooth muscle to contract. Smooth muscle is found all over the body, in the blood vessels, stomach, intestines, stomach, and heart. Bladder muscle is smooth muscle. There is smooth muscle in the prostate too. Here's how an alpha blocker works on your bladder.

Recall in Chapter 1 I explained the inhibitory mechanism that prevents you from wetting your pants and enables you to pee when you're ready. In that chapter, I told you how when your bladder is full, it sends a message via your nerves to your spinal cord and then up to your brain letting you know that your bladder is full, and you'd better find a toilet or someplace in the woods where you can pee. Once in position, unzipped, penis in hand, your brain relays a message that travels down the spinal cord and then via the nerves to the bladder and internal and external sphincters, enabling you to pee.

What's happening in that moment is that several different neurotransmitter chemicals tell the bladder muscle to contract and the sphincter muscles to relax and open. Alpha 1 blockers work at the level of the internal sphincter smooth muscle and help that muscle to relax so that the internal sphincter can more easily open. When they are effective, these drugs can alleviate your symptoms, making it easier to pee and with improved flow, and help the bladder to empty completely so that you don't feel like you have to pee after you just did. Since the bladder empties more completely, it takes longer to fill, which means you won't have to pee so often, or get out of bed multiple times each night, giving you better sleep.

Sometimes that's all that's necessary. But as with all medications, there can be side effects. Because alpha blockers relax smooth muscles, they may affect the smooth muscle elsewhere in the body, not just the bladder. For example, there is smooth muscle in blood vessels, and as those blood vessels relax, your blood pressure can go down, causing you to feel lightheaded or dizzy. You may even faint, though this is rare.

Other possible side effects of alpha blockers are a stuffy nose, and what we call "retrograde ejaculation." During normal ejaculation the bladder neck closes, and semen is expelled through the urethra and out the end of the penis. If the bladder neck doesn't close because the smooth muscle is too relaxed from the alpha blocker, during ejaculation the semen goes backward from the prostatic urethra into the bladder, so nothing comes out of the penis. (That can lead to cloudy urine because the semen is added to the urine the first time you pee after ejaculation.) One possible problem with retrograde ejaculation is it can reduce fertility because you aren't ejaculating, but once the problem is cleared up, you'll be fine. Because most men taking alpha blockers for BPH are older and unconcerned about fertility, so aside from the fact that ejaculation "feels different," this side effect is usually not a concern.

Sometimes when primary care doctors are treating men who have moderate LUTS and moderate bother scores, they will call me because although their patient responded to alpha blockers, they found the side effects intolerable. If that happens to you, ask your doctor if s/he can switch you to a different class of medication that may help. The alternative drugs are called 5 alpha reductase inhibitors, which include finasteride (Proscar) and dutasteride (Avodart). These drugs shrink the prostate (and as an added bonus, they help treat male pattern baldness).

Here's how they work. Testosterone, the male hormone in your body, is responsible for a lot of things—your sex drive (libido), erections, muscle mass and strength, fat metabolism, bone health/mass, the production of red blood cells and sperm, even your behavior. Testosterone also affects the growth of the prostate gland. We know this because we know what happens when there is no testosterone or very low levels of testosterone in men—they have no libido, are frequently impotent, loose muscle mass and strength, and become depressed. Testosterone is converted to dihydrotestosterone by an enzyme called 5 alpha reductase. By blocking this biochemical reaction with finasteride or dutasteride, blood levels of dihydrotestosterone go to zero, while testosterone levels are unchanged. DHT or dihydrotestosterone is also responsible for growth of the prostate gland and seminal vesicles. Take DHT away and the prostate shrinks. We can actually measure the shrinkage using before and after finasteride treatment with transracial ultrasonography.

We also know that both alpha blockers and 5 alpha reductase inhibitors work synergistically. That means that when taken together, their additive effect is greater than the effects of the two drugs combined. In other words, 1 + 1 = 3. These 5 alpha reductase inhibitors are not without side effects and caveats, however. The side effects affect about 10% of men taking Proscar or Avodart, and include a loss of libido, poor or no erections, abnormal ejaculation, weakness, and dizziness. Fortunately, the side effects are usually, but not always, reversible. Understandably, you might be concerned about these side effects, and wonder if you can mitigate them by taking a drug for erectile dysfunction.

That brings us to a discussion about Cialis, a drug that I see constantly advertised on TV for erectile dysfunction (It's part of the same class of drugs called phosphodiesterase 5 inhibitors, which includes

Levitra and Viagra). There are several studies that report improvement of IPSS scores in men taking low dose (5 mg) of Cialis a day. Since Cialis is a drug commonly and effectively (in larger doses) used for erectile dysfunction, those who take it in conjunction with alpha blockers or 5 alpha reductase inhibitors don't have the adverse sexual side effects that you sometimes see with Proscar or Avodart. It would make sense to try it first, right? Well, not exactly. Why? If you look at the medical literature, there is improvement in the IPSS scores, largely a subjective measure, however, flow rates and residual urines, objective measures, did not improve[iii].

Thus, while there are certain patients who do not do well on either alpha blockers or 5 alpha reductase inhibitors, who may benefit from Cialis, it would not be my first, or second choice. But if you are having erectile dysfunction because of Proscar, it's not unreasonable to ask your doctor to prescribe Cialis in low does (5 mg. a day) to help with both ED and LUTS.

There is one other significant factor to consider if taking Proscar or Avodart. These drugs will lower your PSA levels. Because your prostate-specific antigen levels are an early indicator of cancer, your doctor needs to know if you are taking one of these drugs because your PSA will be lower (by 50% or more) than it would be otherwise. This can lead both patient and doctor to a false sense of security, thinking that the risk of clinically significant prostate cancer is much lower than what it really is. (I discuss PSA levels in more detail in Chapter 6.)

Alternative Medicines

Alright, let's say you have some legitimate concerns about taking the medication your physician has recommended or prescribed. You're playing golf or having a beer with some friends, and the talk turns to the problems of aging and you bring up your recent visit to your doctor and why you don't want to take the medicine even if it will help you sleep through the night. That's when one or more of the guys tells you about a better medicine. Something you don't even need a prescription for! It's something you can just buy online!

"Helped me," one of the guys says, "and I haven't had any problem getting it up!"

"Yeah, my brother-in-law is taking something like that," another says, "he said it cured him."

Don't be so sure. If you Google complementary and alternative medicines for treatment of BPH, you'll get 1.5 million hits. There are literally hundreds of products out there promoting "prostate health." This is a multimillion dollar enterprise in the US. In Europe, half of the prescriptions for treatment of BPH are written for complementary and alternative medications. It's certainly possible that some of these products have value, but I am pretty sure some don't. The problem is that many of these products have not been subject to the scrutiny of a formal medical study, which means randomized, prospective, placebo controlled studies. Many of these alternative medicines are no better than placebo, and some have side effects. Any natural remedy that can affect your body therapeutically, can have adverse effects, as well. It's a fallacy that just because something is natural or alternative that it is safe. Keep in mind that there is a fine line between a medicine and a toxin—what can be therapeutic in one dose, can be poisonous in another. Most of the over-the-counter alternative medications that can be purchased online without a prescription, or in your local health food store, but that doesn't make them safe, and it doesn't mean they're regulated and controlled. One review of the literature showed that in small clinical trials for each agent studied, there were mixed results. In other words, some worked, others didn't.

Probably the most popular of the alternative medicines is saw palmetto, which comes from the tree of the same name. Saw palmetto contains a phytosterol (which means it's a type of chemical called a sterol and is related to cholesterol) called beta-sitosterol. Beta-sitosterol is found in a variety of plants and foods in varying amounts, including pumpkin seeds, peanuts, soybeans, pecans, tuna, and certain vegetable oils. One of the problems with saw palmetto may be that the concentration of beta-sitosterol is not high enough to produce a significant effect. Pieter Cohen, a physician and professor of medicine at Harvard Medical School, has studied supplements extensively and concluded that saw palmetto for prostate issues is essentially snake oil—a scam to persuade people to buy a useless product by promising spectacular results. As we know, however, nearly half of the American public is fond of snake oil—we can be easily persuaded by someone who appeals to our emotions, particularly to our fears, as long as they promise to protect us in some way. https://www.consumerreports.org/enlarged-prostate/reasons-to-skip-saw-palmetto-for-enlarged-prostate/

When I set out to do my own research, I felt like I'd crawled down the saw palmetto beta sitosterol rabbit hole. Although the concentration of beta sitosterol is important, it was rarely clear how much was contained in a single pill, while many contained a number of other additives that could potentially be harmful. Without going into a dizzying amount of data and details, suffice it to say that there is extreme variability in the quality and ingredients in these supposed "super prostate" health supplements, and I fear that they are likely to be minimally beneficial at best, potentially harmful at worst. Yet the biggest concern is that by taking these supplements, you might delay early detection of prostate cancer if that were the cause of your enlarged prostate both subjectively and objectively. Subjectively, you could mistakingly assume that the improved symptoms mean the prostate issue has been addressed. Objectively, the supplements could decrease your PSA levels making diagnosis more difficult.

To the extent these supplements do help, what appears to be happening is they might reduce the urinary symptoms, but they do not address the enlarged prostate. In an excellent evidence-based review, beta-sitosterol was said to marginally increase peak flow rate by about 4 cc/sec, reduce residual urine by 25 ml on average, and improve IPSS scores. But there was no evidence that beta-sitosterol reduced the size of the prostate. The reviewer concluded, "The evidence suggests nonglucosidic B-sitosterols improve urinary symptoms and flow measures. Their long term effectiveness, safety and ability to prevent BPH complications are not known.[iv]"

The bottom line is, we don't know how beta-sitosterol works, but some say it acts like a 5 alpha reductase inhibitor. If that's true, why doesn't it decrease the size of the prostate? What effect does it have on PSA? Does dose matter? All of these considerations, and more, would make me more inclined to take something prescribed by my urologist.

There are other caveats to consider if you want to take an alternative medication for your BOO. As I've indicated, the cause of bladder outlet obstructive symptoms is most often from an enlarged and obstructing prostate (BPH), particularly in men over 50. However, this is not always the case. Your prostate does not always have to be enlarged to cause symptoms. It could be inflamed or infected. There may be cancer in your prostate. The problem you are having with decreased urinary flow or blockage may not be due to the prostate at all, but rather from a scar in your urethra, a urethral stricture, as previously mentioned. The problem could also be that your bladder is either inflamed, infected, or cancerous (we discuss bladder cancer in Chapter 9). Even some stones that get lodged in the urethra can cause severe urinary frequency and outlet obstructive symptoms. So if you are going to self-medicate with an alternative medicine concoction, be forewarned—you might be treating the symptoms, but missing the cause of those symptoms to your detriment.

The second concern is that these alternative medications like saw palmetto are not regulated by the FDA. That means you don't know whether what the label says is actually true, both in terms of the actual ingredients in each pill, and the amount/concentration of each ingredient. (One study in Florida analyzed six brands of saw palmetto and found that half of them contained less than 20 percent of the amount stated on the label[v].)

Nor do you know whether the claims made about the ingredients are accurate. These products are not subjected to the same scrutiny and testing as FDA approved drugs, they are often mislabeled, and many are made in other countries with lax standards and quality control. There can be far less of the active ingredient than what is stated on the label. Some of the "wonder drugs" may also contain real active drugs, such as Viagra, in them that aren't mentioned on the label so that the drugs can produce a response. These drugs are in doses that are not regulated and can produce serious side effects. They could also interact with medications you are taking—which is one of many reasons why it's imperative that if you do take such supplements or alternative medications, you let your physician know about it. Don't withhold the information because you fear judgment. Your doctor needs to know what you're putting into your body in order to help you.

You also need to take into consideration the placebo effect. Several of these alternative medications, particularly saw palmetto, have been subjected to empirical testing comparing their effects to placebos. These studies show no difference in improvement of symptoms between groups of men taking placebos compared to men taking saw palmetto.[vi] If you are thinking you are saving money (a bottle of 250 saw palmetto pills can be had for as little as $25) by avoiding doctor visits and prescription medicine, think again. Your symptoms would likely improve with a daily sugar pill. By not addressing the problem correctly, delay in the correct diagnosis and treatment may make the problem worse than it already is. So what can you do, besides take costly medications with serious side effects? Though I don't want to discourage you from taking prescribed medications (you should if you need to), the good news is that there are a few things you can do that might help you.

If your symptoms are mild, and you want to avoid taking prescription medications, you you can do some things to improve matters:

- Cut back on drinks between dinner and bedtime, especially alcoholic and caffeinated beverages which can act like diuretics and increase your need to pee;
- Limit the use of antihistamines and decongestants, because these drugs have an affect on the smooth muscle of the bladder and internal sphincter and can make it more difficult to pee;
- If you take a diuretic for high blood pressure, ask your doctor about changing the time you take it, reducing the dose, or trying a different drug.

Minimally-Invasive Procedures

Sometimes medication doesn't resolve the problem. If that's the case, your urologist may discuss a minimally invasive procedure (MIP) to correct the problem. There are a number of such procedures, so let's start with those that can done in the urologist's office under local anesthesia (meaning you will be sedated and the area numb, but you will remain awake). These procedures usually work best when the size of the prostate is less than 30 or 40 grams (determined by ultrasound). You might opt for a minimally invasive procedure because there is faster recovery and fewer risks and complications compared to the more invasive procedures. As you will see, the evolution of these innovative minimally invasive procedures has been dramatic.

Transurethral Microwave Thermotherapy (TUMT)

A common MIP, and one that I have performed many times, is the Transurethral Microwave Thermotherapy (TUMT). After your urethra has been numbed with a local anesthetic, a special catheter is inserted through the urethra and into the bladder. The catheter is hooked up to a machine that sends microwave energy and heat through the catheter and prostate. At the same time, the part of the catheter in the urethra has a balloon that inflates and dilates the urethra at the same time the microwave is heating and destroying prostate tissue. The temperature in the bladder and rectum is monitored throughout the procedure to ensure these organs are not injured. Your doctor will perform two cycles of this procedure. The procedure is tolerated well, and though two cycles are done back to back, they take less than 45 minutes total. While initially effective, many men find the improved stream and decrease in residual urine doesn't last beyond a few months. Consequently, the procedure has largely been abandoned and replaced with newer procedures that work better.

Urolift

Another common MIP treatment for BPH is a Urolift. To understand how the procedure works, think of the bladder as a hollowed out small grapefruit with the pulp removed, attached to a tangerine—your prostate. Now imagine a straw—representing your urethra—going through the pulp of the tangerine. That is essentially how your bladder, prostate and urethra fit together, your pee goes through the straw, which goes through the tangerine pulp. With a Urolift, a long scope is inserted into the urethra, spring like implant placed from inside the prostate (from inside the straw), thru the pulp of the tangerine and exited through to the outside of the tangerine orange. A bolster sits on each end of the spring-implant,. So there is an outer bolster outside the "rind of the tangerine" and an inner bolster inside the prostatic urethra "the straw". The prostate tissue is compressed or squeezed between the two bolsters, effectively compressing the prostate tissue (pulp of the tangerine) creating more room for the urine to pass through the prostate. The procedure works best on small and medium prostates.

Now back to that tangerine (prostate) and hollowed out grapefruit (bladder). Larger prostates may require more than two or even four spring-like implants. Depending on the length of the part of the straw going through the prostate, or the length of the prostate itself as measured from bladder to the external sphincter, which is the other end of the prostate or prostatic apex, the end opposite the bladder. As with any medical procedure, Urolift has its advantages and disadvantages. The advantages of the Urolift procedure are that a catheter is often not required following the procedure, sexual dysfunction and incontinence are uncommon, and usual activities can be resumed in a few days. But there are definite limitations and disadvantages to the procedure.

Limitations of Urolift relate to the overall size and length of the prostate. It only works on prostates less than than 6.5 cm long (about the length of a man's ring finger). If the prostate is long, then multiple needle/bolster placements are needed and the results may not be as good when compared to an average length prostate. And, if the prostate is really large in width (from the outside of the right lobe to the outside of the left lobe), the spring-like implants won't be long enough to be properly placed. These measurements are easily determined by doing a transrectal ultrasound of the prostate.

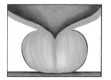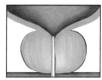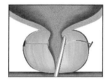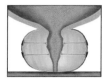

Uro-lift Procedure

Nor will Urolift work as well if there is a large median lobe of the prostate. Your prostate has two "lobes," through which the urethra passes (imagine that tangerine again, with each half of the tangerine pulp a lobe, right and left, on each side of the straw). These lobes are what constrict the urethra. Sometimes, however, a median lobe of the prostate develops as well, resting like a golf ball inside the bladder and between the two lobes. Many men have no median lobe at all, while others can have a fairly large one. If you do have a median lobe (diagnosed by cystoscopy), a Urolift will likely be unsuccessful.

Urolift can be quite effective, but there are potential problems. Though the procedure should not be painful, the first few days post-procedure can be uncomfortable, a burning sensation when urinating and some bleeding in the urine or noted in the underwear. Because you are given antibiotics following the procedure, there is an unlikely chance you could develop a UTI. The procedure is effective, however, and follow-up has thus far shown that it can lasts up to four years.

Rezum

One relatively new procedure that can be done in your urologist's office or an outpatient facility is Rezum. Though I have never performed one because the procedure was introduced after my retirement in

2014, a man I golf with succinctly described the procedure as having his prostate "steam cleaned." With Rezum, a thin (4mm), rigid cystoscope is passed into the prostate via the urethra. A special needle is inserted under vision into the pulp of the tangerine. Steam is then injected through the needle into the targeted obstructing tissue of the prostate in nine-second bursts. The water vapor gets into the cells, killing them. Basically, what happens is the solid part of the prostate is turned to liquid and the liquid is then resorbed, resulting in an average decrease of 30% of the prostate's volume.

Rezum has been endorsed by the AUA for treatment of BPH and has been found to be effective in lowering IPSS scores, significantly improving flow rates, and reducing residual urine volume. Only 5% of patients require further treatment. What's more, there is minimal bleeding, and sexual side effects, such as impotence and/or ejaculatory dysfunction (retrograde ejaculation) are less common when compared to more invasive procedures.

Most patients tolerate the procedure with oral sedation and local anesthesia (Novacain jelly in the urethra). Some patients will better tolerate the procedure if a nerve block is done in the same technique that we use prior to prostate biopsy using transrectal ultrasound guidance. About ten percent of patients undergoing the procedure will require intravenous sedation. One disadvantage when compared to Urolift, however, is that you may require a catheter for a few days.

Because the procedure is so new, we don't have data on the long-term effectiveness of the procedure, but we do know that after two to three years, there has been no need for additional treatment.

But not all men and not all prostates are good candidates for Re-zum. If the prostate volume is too great, or if there is a median lobe, the procedure won't work as well.

If your urologist is recommending this procedure, ask him or her how many of these procedures they have done (because it is so new, they may be relatively inexperienced with the procedure). What kind of anesthesia do they recommend? Will you need a catheter after the procedure and if so, how long? What kinds of complications (such as bleeding, pain, scar tissue formation anywhere along the urinary tract, or sexual dysfunction) have their patients had? You should also ask about the size of your prostate. If it is less than 80 cubic centimeters, and you don't have a median lobe, you're a candidate for Urolift or Rezum. But if you do have a median lobe or your prostate is greater than 100 cubic centimeters, you are most likely going to need a more invasive procedure.

Aquablation

Another recent invasive innovation is Aquablation, which delivers a jet of saline that destroys the tissue (think of the pulp of the tangerine as the tissue you want to remove). Like Rezum and Urolift, the proce-dure is done through the urethra, but uses ultrasound imaging to ex-actly calibrate and direct the saline jet. The procedure requires gen-eral or spinal anesthesia. The average time of resection is about 30 min, which for a large gland is half the time required for a TURP. Aquablation was approved by the FDA in 2018.

An ultrasound probe is placed into the rectum and a scope in the urethra is attached to a robotic arm. The robotic arm + the scope, the high velocity saline jet, and the ultrasound are all linked via computer to deliver the saline directly to the tissue. It's reported to be quick procedure, just seven to ten minutes, yet requires a night in the hospital and may require electrocautery to control minor bleeding. You will need to have a catheter for 1-3 days after the procedure, and there is the slight risk of post operative bleeding and scar tissue forming, but bleeding should resolve within a few days and scar tissue (scar of the bladder neck at the bladder prostate junction - bladder neck contracture, or scar in the urethra itself - urethral stricture). The good news is that early clinical studies report few problems with erectile and ejaculation dysfunction.

Aquablation is a very promising technique that has been slow to gain popularity, primarily because the Covid pandemic limited exposure to the procedure to clinical urologists who could be recommending it to patients. The same is true for Rezum. It's my opinion that the combination of ultrasound guided resection combined with direct vision resection, or in the case of aquablation, robot and computer guided resection, is the way of the near future. The safety and execution of the operation is not as dependent on the skill or experience of the urologist when compared to a TURP, or as we'll discuss next, HoLEP. Like HoLEP, aquablation works well for large prostates (> 70 grams), has good outcomes, and few complications.

I repeat, if your urologist recommends one of these newer procedures, ask him/her about their experience has been with each procedure, how have they turned out, what complications have they seen, as well as any other available alternatives. If you are still uncomfortable, it's reasonable to seek another opinion.

Transurethral Needle Ablation of the Prostate (TUNA)

Another less popular minimally-invasive procedure is the Transurethral Needle Ablation of the Prostate (TUNA). In this procedure, needles are inserted in the prostate to heat and destroy the tissue. This procedure is not one I nor many doctors recommend, because the other procedures are preferred.

Prostate Artery Embolization

One last procedure a bit more invasive than these others but still considered "minimally invasive" is prostate artery embolization. This procedure is only advised for patients who are not candidates for anything else, and is performed by interventional radiologists—physicians trained in radiology who do procedures in addition to interpreting imaging studies. Under fluroscopic (x-ray) guidance, the radiologist threads a wire into a large artery (usually your leg). The wire is guided into the artery that feeds the prostate. A catheter is then placed over the wire. The radiologist will inject dye to into the catheter to map the blood supply to the prostate. Once s/he has identified the blood supply, a solution containing "microspheres" (tiny microscopic plastic beads) is injected through the catheter to occlude the blood supply to the prostate. By depriving the prostate of its' blood supply, the cells die and the prostate shrinks.

As frightening as the procedure might sound, it's actually fairly simple and has fewer side effects than invasive procedures. The most common side effect is temporary urinary retention (incomplete emptying of the bladder). My greatest caution, however, is that you want an experienced radiologist performing the procedure. This is a rare procedure and reserved only if you are at high risk of bleeding (because you are on blood thinners or won't accept a blood transfusion for religious reasons), or because you may have other medical problems making you a poor candidate for anything else.

Invasive Procedures

Now that you know your options for a less invasive procedure, what happens if your doctor recommends a more invasive procedure, one performed under general anesthesia (where you are not conscious) or spinal anesthesia (where you can't feel anything from the waist down)? There are several reasons your physician may recommend such a procedure, and it's reasonable for you to ask why this particular procedure and not one of the alternatives. It may be that his/her experience with less invasive procedures has been limited or unsatisfactory in producing good outcomes. If that's the case, you might want to consider getting a second opinion, because it may be better to have a less invasive procedure *if you are a good candidate for it*. Another reason may be that you've already had a minimally-invasive procedure, but it didn't improve your flow rate or decrease your residual urine. If that's the case, you might need a more invasive procedure. Generally speaking, invasive procedures are more definitive in relieving the obstruction and work better than minimally-invasive options and drugs. Or it may be the case, and often is, that other issues such as infections, the size of your prostate, the anatomy of your prostate (such as a large median lobe, for example), or a large residual volume of urine, make a more invasive procedure more likely to produce a good result.

Whatever the reason, you are entitled to an explanation for why your urologist is recommending a more invasive procedure which requires either a spinal block or general anesthetic. This is a situation in which shared decision making can be valuable. You and your urologist can discuss the alternative procedures and the risks and benefits of each.

There are good reasons to consider a more invasive procedure: The obstruction could be causing so much pressure that your kidneys are unable to work properly; an enlarged prostate can cause significant bleeding; the obstruction has caused a bladder stone to form; if you've been having recurring UTI's due to the obstruction and a lot of urine still in your bladder after you pee; or if despite other treatments, you still can't pee. Sometimes the obstruction is so severe that you are unable to pee at all. This is called urinary retention and requires temporary catheter drainage or intermittent catheterization to empty the bladder. When this happens, a more invasive treatment is usually required.

Let's take a look at the most common of these procedures, all of which have the goal of removing the obstructing prostate tissue, either completely or partially. Think of it as removing the pulp of the tangerine, while leaving the rind intact. These operations are done to remove benign, noncancerous prostate tissue, whereas surgery for prostate cancer requires removal of the entire prostate, the seminal vesicles, and the ejaculatory ducts, with reconstruction of the urinary tract to attach the bladder neck directly to the urethra.

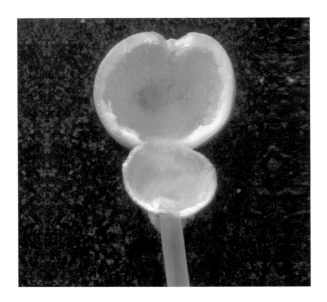

Prostate Anatomy After TURP, HoLEP, Supra-pubic prostatectomy.

Large hollowed orange = bladder. Smaller orange with pulp removed is resected prostate, straw is the urethra, note, external sphincter not part of the model, but I used a large paper clip at the junction of the straw and smaller orange to demonstrate this

Transurethral Resection of the Prostate (TURP)

Transurethral resection of the prostate, commonly called TURP (or transurethral prostatectomy) is the most common form of surgery for BPH. If you have a TURP, you will be hospitalized for one to two days, though there are some urologists who perform TURPs as an outpatient procedure. There are two types of TURPs, monopolar and bipolar, and both are performed under spinal or general anesthesia. In a TURP, the surgeon inserts an instrument known as a resectoscope into your urethra, which has a wire loop on one end. Electrical current (mono or bipolar) is sent to this loop, which resects and cauterizes the prostate tissue, removing the blockage and enabling you to pee freely again.

The resectoscope is placed through the penile urethra into the prostatic urethra (the straw). The image of the inside of the prostate is displayed on a monitor. A wire loop is moved back and forth, cutting small pieces of prostate tissue (the pulp of the tangerine). The tissue "chips" are irrigated into the bladder while the urologist moves the wire loop. Simultaneously s/he can stop the bleeding with the loop because the current passing into the loop cauterizes the tissue. With a mono-polar loop, the irrigation fluid is water, sorbitol, or glycine. With bipolar loops, normal saline can be used, which is safer. The reason a bipolar TURP is safer is due to the difference in the fluid used to irrigate. If a vein is open during the procedure, the irrigation fluid gets into the bloodstream. Water, sorbitol, and glycine can cause problems when this happens, whereas saline does not.

I started doing bipolar transurethral surgery for prostate and bladder problems 15 years before my retirement in 2014 and it was a game changer. I stopped doing the mono-polar TURP altogether and used bipolar energy exclusively. The bipolar loops were smaller than the mono-polar and the TURP took slightly longer to perform. But by using a normal saline solution for irrigation the procedure much safer. I found the bipolar procedure to be elegant, as if completing an underwater internal human sculpture done through some guy's penis could be called elegant. Adopting the bipolar procedure was like driving a Tesla or Porsche after driving a Toyota Corolla all those years.

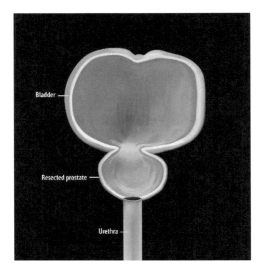

Prostate Anatomy After TURP, HoLEP, suprapubic prostatectomy

Transurethral Incision of the Prostate (TUIP) - If the bladder neck (where the bladder and prostate join) is "tight", and lesser invasive and faster method of treating obstruction is simply incising the bladder neck/prostate. If you look at the bladder neck as if it were a clock, incisions are made at 5 or 7 o'clock, or both. No tissue is removed. The complication of retrograde ejaculation occurs less often if only one side is incised. This is a reasonable procedure for some patients, particularly those men who have responded to alpha blockers but don't like the side effects.

Another advance in medicine has been in the use of lasers. Lasers have many applications in many fields of medicine. In urology, various types of lasers are used for treating problems in the kidney, ureter, bladder, prostate, and urethra. Lasers are helpful in treating benign and malignant conditions, stones, and scar tissue. When it comes to BPH, lasers can remove the pulp of the tangerine and leave the rind.

Some urologists will recommend using a laser first before a TURP, because there is less risk of bleeding, and it can be performed as an outpatient procedure. I performed several dozen "laser TURPs" or "Green light laser TURPs." Nonetheless, I abandoned using lasers for TURPs because I was not satisfied with the way things looked when I was done. Also, some of the patients had more postoperative pain with urination after the procedure. I didn't think the amount of intra-operative or post operative bleeding was less than a bipolar TURP. But if you are considering laser surgery for your BPH, here's a summary of the HoLEP procedure which your urologist might recommend.

Holmium Laser Enucleation of the Prostate (HoLEP)

When the prostate is extremely large (the size of a tennis ball) or over 80 grams, a few skilled urologists prefer an enucleation procedure (enucleation means to remove something; think of it as removing the pulp of the tangerine intact, rather than taking the tissue out in bits and pieces) called HoLEP.

HoLEP is a very specialized procedure, one done in a hospital under general or spinal anesthesia. The procedure takes two to three hours, during which a urologist inserts a holmium laser fiber through a scope in your urethra. S/he then uses a Holmium laser fiber to separate the pulp of the prostate from the inner capsule or rind. The whole pulp of the prostate is pushed into the bladder and an instrument called a morselizer is passed through the scope and grinds up the pulp. The "morselized" tissue is then irrigated out of the bladder. This is a difficult procedure to learn and these days is something learned in fellowship training, or from a urologist who has a great deal of experience.

There are other invasive procedures usually reserved for very large prostates or conditions in which there is more going on than just BPH. For example, if there are bladder stones or a bladder diverticulum (an out pouching that's either congenital or more often caused by BPH), it's advantageous to take care of all the problems at the same time. That is, remove the stone(s), relieve the obstruction from the large prostate, and/or remove the diverticulum. Sometimes this can be done through the urethra using scopes, lasers, or special tools to break up stones using ultrasound energy. Some urologists would prefer taking care of the problem through an incision in the abdomen, then bladder. BPH tissue removed in this manner is called a suprapubic prostatectomy. These procedures can be done through laparoscopes alone or robot-assisted laparoscopes. Much of the decision depends on surgeon preference, experience, and outcomes. If this is you, know that it's okay to ask about alternatives, risks, and benefits.

One last remark about invasive procedures. If you are one of those unfortunate individuals who is in acute or chronic urinary retention, which means you are unable to empty your bladder at all, you DO NOT want to have one of these procedures unless your urologist is sure that your bladder muscle (called the detrussor) works. There are times when a person goes into urinary retention. The bladder muscle is stretched beyond a point where the muscle fibers don't work. This can be temporary or permanent. Your urologist can do a simple test (called a cystometrogram) to tell if your bladder has recovered and the muscle is working. If the bladder muscle has been so severely stretched, or if there is a neurological cause for the urinary retention (a condition called a "flaccid bladder"), then no matter how effective the procedure is in removing the blockage, by whatever means, the bladder still won't work, and you will still be unable to empty and still require catheterization. A severely stretched bladder requires at least 7-10 days to recover. Your bladder needs to heal and rest, and you need to be sure of that before you have an invasive procedure to remove the inner part of your prostate.

Conclusion

What's Best for You? Like most things in medicine, there is no blanket formula or simple answer to help you with your enlarged obstructing prostate. Every prostate and every man's slow stream (plus other symptoms) deserve to be individualized before embarking on treatment. Treatment decisions are based on the severity of your symptoms, the size of your enlarged prostate, your lifestyle considerations (such as how much time and help you have to recover and your personal concerns), and whether your enlarged prostate is causing more harmful issues, such as urinary retention, kidney failure, bladder stones, bladder diverticula, infections, or bleeding. The decision is also based on which possible side-effects you are comfortable with, or not. Many of these procedures are based on the training, skill, and experience of the surgeon, so a shared decision making conversation will help. With all that in mind, go forth and pee strong.

CHAPTER 6

Should I Get a PSA?

Whether I'm on the golf course, enjoying a casual get together with friends, or find myself seated on a jet engaged in a conversation with a total stranger, once a man knows I'm a urologist, one of the most common questions that I'm asked is, "Tell me doc, should I get a PSA?"

A PSA is an inexpensive blood test that identifies levels of a prostate specific antigen, which is a marker for prostate cancer. Now, you might think detecting any sign of cancer is a good thing, but as you'll see, the answer isn't simple, which is why my first response is usually, "Why do you ask?"

The replies I receive range from "Just wondering. It's pretty controversial, right?" to "My doctor says it's not recommended anymore, is he right?" And of course, there's the ever-popular, "I Googled PSA testing and there were 27 million results!" a response that is inevitably followed by some irrational fear that having the test will end life as you know it. In short, the information floating around on the internet about PSA is not designed to inform you, but to unnecessarily alarm you, while half of what you read is utter nonsense and the other half too confusing to make sense of. That's why so many people get their information from their friends.

"I know a guy who had a PSA and his doctor sent him to a urologist, the urologist did a biopsy, he bled when he peed for two weeks, and the biopsy turned out negative! He went through all that misery for nothing!"

"I know a guy who had a PSA five years ago, his doctor told him it was normal, and he had nothing to worry about, and now he's got really bad prostate cancer. What good did it do him?"

"I know a guy who had a slightly abnormal PSA. A urologist did a biopsy and found a small spot of cancer. The urologist said it was slow growing, but he should have it removed anyway. So he had one of those robot surgeries to remove his prostate, and now he can't get it up and he wears diapers!"

I've heard so many "I know a guy" stories, and I don't doubt such scenarios do happen. The problem with these stories though is that anecdotes are the worst way to inform yourself, much less to base an informed medical decision on—especially one in which your life might depend.

So What Exactly is PSA?

To understand the controversy, let's first understand what a Prostate Specific Antigen (PSA) actually is. An antigen is a protein, and the prostate specific antigen is made by benign and malignant prostate cells (with some rare exceptions, which we don't need to go into here). PSA is found inside the tissue of the prostate, in blood, and in places where cancer cells spread to outside the prostate (such as bones and lymph nodes, which we discuss in the next chapter).

The higher the PSA level, the more of the antigen there is in the blood. The more PSA there is, the more likely it is that there are more benign or malignant prostate cells producing it. If you have a high PSA, it doesn't mean that you have cancer, it just means there's a greater statistical probability that there may be some malignant prostate cancer cells either in your prostate, or even outside your prostate (usually in the bones or lymph nodes), or both.

Because all men with prostates have a certain level of PSA in their bodies as they get older, every man of a certain age has a *unique* PSA, and that PSA is associated with a statistical risk of having or not having cancer. Our unique risk changes over time. We also know that as we get older, PSA increases, whether we have cancer in the prostate or not. BPH, discussed in the last chapter, leads to an increase in PSA. Chronic inflammation of the prostate and other factors, discussed further on, can also increase PSA levels.

Most labs report PSA levels as "normal" if they fall below 4.0. Yet there is no such thing as a "normal" PSA. Every PSA is associated with a risk of having prostate cancer, and every man's PSA is unique to him. So, with those points in mind, there really is no normal. What's important is how that specific PSA level defines the risk that every unique man has of having prostate cancer, based on a range of variables.

Before I dive into the details of PSA and how to use PSA to assess prostate cancer risk, let me tell a couple of stories of my own, to show you why interpreting these levels can be lifesaving.

Five Men, Five Different Outcomes

When I met him, "Scott" (as we'll call him) was a well-known 48 year old African American athlete. After retiring from his professional career, Scott coached a U.S. Olympic team and a college team that won an NCAA Division I National Championship. He was nationally revered as one of the best coaches in his sport, and had come to me for a routine matter when I asked him, "When was your last PSA?" His answer astounded me.

Not only had he never had a PSA, something in itself that wasn't surprising, he had never even been asked about one, nor had any physician ever done a rectal exam to check his prostate. He had been insured, and been seen by countless doctors given his profession, but never had there been any discussion about a basic screening test most men his age routinely undergo—a disturbing reality for far too many African Americans who do not always receive the same standards of care that caucasian males do.

By the time I did the test, his PSA was over 100 and his prostate was rock hard and very abnormal. The biopsy and subsequent testing revealed he had prostate cancer which had advanced to metastatic cancer—meaning the cancer had spread beyond his prostate to other tissues, bones and lymph nodes. There was nothing we could do to save his life, the best we could hope for was prolonging it and alleviating his discomfort. Three years later, after multiple surgeries, hormone ablation therapy, standard and experimental chemotherapy, Scott died. He was just 51 years old.

I'd grown close to Scott in those three years, and his death was one of the saddest I've encountered in my career, made all the more difficult to accept because it was probably preventable. Had Scott received a rectal exam and a PSA screening, in all likelihood he'd be alive today.

There's another patient I want to tell you about before we get into the nitty-gritty of PSA, because his case, and those of his sons, illustrates another important point about PSA—each person's PSA is only one of several variables that must be considered before taking further action, and each story is unique.

"John" was a 67 year old physician who had seen his internist because he was having problems peeing. He was getting up three to five times a night to pee, peeing frequently throughout the day with a slow stream, and feeling like he couldn't empty his bladder. His internist told him he had a "very big" prostate and put him on an alpha blocker and finasteride to shrink the prostate (see Chapter 4 for more information about these medications). John asked his doctor about getting a PSA, and his doctor shrugged it off, telling him, "I don't believe in them, they're not accurate and the USPTF (United States Preventative Task Force) says we shouldn't do them anyway. Besides, your prostate's so big that the PSA will be elevated anyway." With that, John didn't pursue the matter further, confident his physician's advice was sound.

Unfortunately, the medications did little to resolve his symptoms, and within a year, John returned to his internist. By now his urinary problems were secondary to the pain he felt in his back. His right leg had swollen to five times the size of his left. He had massive pitting edema, meaning there was so much excess fluid in his right leg that it would not spring back when pressed, leaving "pits" in his flesh.

Given these alarming symptoms, he was referred to a urologist who ordered a PSA—the first PSA John had ever had, even though the test had already been around for 15 years. The results were startling—John's PSA was over 200! Subsequent tests determined he had metastatic prostate cancer that had spread to his pelvic lymph nodes that drain the right leg (which explained the swelling, as the tumors blocked the lymph drainage). The cancer had also spread to several of his bones, including his spine. To control his pain from the cancer in his bones, he underwent radiation therapy, followed by chemotherapy, and he was put on hormone ablation therapy. The treatments worked for about a year, but ultimately failed. Two years after his diagnosis, John died. I can't help but imagine what his last years may have been like if, when he had asked his doctor about a PSA, his doctor had given him a different answer, such as "Well, you do have a remarkably large prostate, and you are 67 years old. Let's do a PSA and take it from there."

John's story doesn't end with his death. John had five adult sons. After their father's death, they each began getting their own PSAs. His oldest son began getting PSAs at the age of 55. Doing so provided him a base level, and when it shot up from 2.0 to 5.0, he had a biopsy. The biopsy revealed he had prostate cancer, evaluated as "moderate" on what we call the Gleason scale (discussed in more detail in Chapter 7). He elected radiation therapy, and twelve years later, when I last spoke with him, he was effectively cancer free (I say "effectively" because we do not consider cancer to be cured until 15 years after treatment.) He was at that time receiving annual PSA screenings, and his levels remained less than 1, which is considered an excellent response to radiation. In this case, John's eldest son was wise to get a PSA test, which may have saved his life. He was between the ages of 40 and 75, and his father had died from prostate cancer. Those two factors suggested a PSA was worthwhile—as it proved to be for two of his brothers. However, for one the PSA testing turned out to have a different outcome.

John's second to eldest son started getting PSAs when he turned 50. Like his elder brother, six years his senior, he was in the age range recommended by most urologists for PSAs, and both his father and brother had had prostate cancer. Initially, his PSA level was "normal", but over time it rose to over 4.0, what labs regard as the "abnormal" level. He had a biopsy, which did not show any cancer. A year later, however, his PSA had risen even more, so he had a second biopsy, again negative. Two years passed, and his PSA continued to rise. His urologist was concerned, and thus subjected him to 50 biopsies all done at the same time under general anesthesia, something called "saturation" biopsies. This time, prostate cancer was detected.

The biopsies, however, caused a severe infection, and he ended up in the ICU for several days being treated for sepsis. He recovered, but the severe infection left him reluctant to have anything done to treat his cancer, in the hope that it would be slow growing. Two more years passed and as his PSAs continued to rise, he finally decided to be treated. Given his brother's good response to radiation, he opted for the same. He had a good response, initially, but then his PSA began to climb again. Further tests revealed the prostate cancer had metastasized to his bones. He was treated with hormone ablation therapy, and after a year, his PSA was undetectable. But the side effects of the treatment had made him miserable, so given the decrease in his PSA, hormone ablation was stopped. I wish I could tell you that his story ended well, but the last I heard, his PSA was rising again at a fast rate, and as I write this, he is receiving chemotherapy to control metastatic cancer.

Should he have gotten a PSA? Yes. But in his case, the biopsies done for a rising PSA produced something we call a false negative— they indicated there was no cancer, which probably was not the case. His persistently rising PSA levels indicated something was wrong. Because he became septic after the saturation biopsies he opted not to be treated for the cancer when it was finally diagnosed. Might the outcome have been different if he'd never had a PSA in the first place, and thus, not had the biopsies? Probably not, because he still did have cancer. And one indicator of that cancer was his rising PSA. It was his decision to delay treatment for cancer that ultimately spread. Currently, things are different. A man who now has a PSA that shows he is at high risk for having prostate cancer, yet has negative biopsies, will likely *not* have saturation biopsies, but a special MRI of the prostate called a "multi detector MRI. In this case, the MRI would have likely shown an abnormality that could be specifically targeted and biopsied.

The youngest of John's five sons began getting PSAs at age 52, based on his father's and two older brother's history. When he turned 55, his PSA had increased from 2.0 to 4.1, so his urologist recommended a biopsy. Three of the 12 biopsies showed cancer, moderately differentiated (or intermediate risk), like his eldest brother. After watching what had happened with his father and two of his four brothers, he elected a robotic radical prostatectomy. He wanted that cancer out of there asap. Upon microscopic examination of the specimen, the pathologist noted at the cut edge of the prostate, what we call, "margin positive disease") his physician decided not to treat him with radiation therapy, but to just keep an eye on his PSA. As of this writing, he is five years post-surgery, and his PSA remains undetectable. What's more, despite the prostatectomy, he is neither incontinent nor impotent. Best of all, he is alive.

These three stories show that determining your PSA levels can save your life. PSA is not a diagnostic test, as biopsies are. PSA is a simple, inexpensive blood test. That is all. PSA does not tell you if you have cancer—it provides an indicator that may mean something is going on. To diagnose cancer, you usually need a biopsy, an MRI, or both. And yes, biopsies can cause infections and bleeding in fewer than 2% of men who undergo prostate biopsy, but given a choice between a treatable infection and cancer, which would you prefer?

Before and After PSA

When I started my urology residency in 1979 at Oregon Health Sciences University in Portland, we did very few radical prostatectomies (complete removal of the prostate). That was because by the time a man has symptoms of prostate cancer (and these can be local symptoms or symptoms from the spread of the cancer), it's usually too late to cure it. In the late 70s and early 80s, not many lives were saved. We could though slow the spread of cancer with "hormone therapy, either by castration or estrogens. 95% of testosterone (male hormone) comes from the testicles. Huggins and Hodges (University of Chicago) showed in 1941 that castration resulted in slower growth or temporary disappearance of prostate cancer. Dr. Huggins won the Nobel Prize in medicine for this work in 1966, and Dr Hodges was chairman of the Department of Urology at Oregon Health Science University in 1979 when I started the urology residency there. They also showed that estrogen (oral or intravenous) had a similar affect on prostate cancer as castration. As you can imagine, neither of these treatments—castration or estrogen therapy—would be high on the list of most men's treatment options, but there just wasn't much else we could do to treat men with metastatic prostate cancer.

At that time, the diagnosis of localized prostate cancer (cancer which has not spread beyond the prostate) was made by a digital rectal exam (DRE). It was rare to diagnose localized prostate cancer because most men did not have any symptoms, and it was difficult to feel a small nodule, especially for a general practitioner or internist who lacks the experience of a urologist in detecting such tiny lumps.

If such a nodule was detected, the man would undergo a crude blind biopsy through the rectum or perineum (the space between the scrotum and anus). By "blind" I mean that the biopsy was not done with the aid of today's trans-rectal ultrasound or MRI imaging. Instead, a biopsy needle was guided by an index finger into the rectum. As you can imagine, such a procedure was not pleasant, and could result in mistakes, but it was all we had.

As for markers, the only marker we had that there might be cancer was a blood test called acid phosphatase. Acid phosphatase is an enzyme made in a variety of organs—the prostate, bone marrow, spleen and liver. Given its presence in so many organs, it was only used as an indicator of advanced or metastatic prostate disease. A "normal" level didn't mean much, because the cancer could be in the prostate, even beyond it, and still the levels could be normal. By the time a patient had an elevated acid phosphatase level, it was an ominous sign—it usually meant stage III or IV.

We commonly found prostate cancer when a man had significant symptoms. He'd come to us with problems peeing and have a rock hard prostate. Often, by the time they came to us they already had symptoms of cancer in the bone (back pain, hip pain, rib pain, pelvic pain) or lymph nodes (swelling in one or both legs, or other 'blockages' from cancerous lymph nodes).We saw very little early stage prostate cancer when I first started out. In fact, I only witnessed two radical prostatectomies in my entire three year residency in urology. I saw, instead, a lot of castrations. That's because most of the prostate cancer I saw was advanced and/or metastatic

cancer.

At the V.A. hospital in Portland in the early 80s, it wasn't at all unusual for urology residents and attending staff to care for men who had fought in WWII, Korea or Vietnam. More than half of these men were diagnosed with advanced prostate cancer that had spread to their bones or lymph nodes. Cancer in the bones can be extremely painful, and sometimes results in what we call a "pathologic fracture." The bones break spontaneously because of the cancer. Worse, when bone cancer involves the spine, the tumors can compress the spinal cord and cause paralysis. These men were treated with intravenous estrogen and radiation to the involved bones. Most did not survive beyond one or two years. Many died excruciating deaths—all because their cancer hadn't been caught early. Then along came PSA and all that changed.

When PSA was discovered in the early eighties, it was a game changer. I started practice at Kaiser in Portland, Oregon in 1982. We started using PSA as a "screening tool" for prostate cancer in 1986. We found that it was much more sensitive and even more specific than acid phosphatase. The more we used PSA, the more excited we got. PSA not only helped us to detect cancer much earlier, before it had spread beyond the prostate, it also enabled us to more accurately assess patient responses to treatments for prostate cancer.

We began diagnosing prostate cancers before we could even feel them and before they had a chance to spread. I went from doing castrations or putting men on a new hormone ablation therapy for metastatic prostate cancer called Lupron, to doing two radical prostatectomies a week (recall that I had done only two during my entire residency). Our "cure rates" (based on an immeasurable PSA after complete removal) were well above 90%, *if* the cancer was confined to the prostate. This was a quantum change in the way we treated prostate cancer. Instead of 50% of men presenting with advanced or metastatic prostate cancer, only 10% of men presenting with prostate cancer had metastatic disease. We were convinced that PSA was profoundly necessary for early detection of prostate cancer, and that it was saving lives and preventing life altering morbidity.

But there was a problem. Not all doctors who weren't urologist felt the same enthusiasm for PSA, or PSA "screening". Some felt that urologists were taking way too many prostates out of men with small slow growing cancers that would never cause them any harm whatsoever, and that the treatments were causing more harms than benefits.

So, in 2008, the U.S. Preventative Task Force (USPTF) advised *against* using PSA as a screening test. Almost overnight, men stopped having their PSAs checked, doctors stopped recommending them. Soon I found myself debating the "controversy" of PSA, and PSA "screening" (the reason I put "screening" in quotes is because I prefer to think of using PSA as an "early detection" tool - the difference is important). I've been embroiled in this controversy since 1986.

In over 35 years of practice, I cared for thousands of men with prostate cancer, and did tens of thousands of prostate biopsies on men, some of whom turned out not to have prostate cancer. If I am an expert on anything, PSA-based testing for early detection of prostate cancer is in my wheelhouse. So why the controversy, and did those all those men who had negative biopsies have them for no reason? Let's talk about the controversy, the nuances of PSA testing for early detection, and why I feel that PSA is still a very useful tool for saving lives and preventing significant morbidity. Hopefully this discussion will help you answer the question "Should I get a PSA?"//

The USPTF Recommendations of PSA for Cancer Screening

The controversy starts with the USPTF (US Preventative Task Force) in 2008. The USPTF studies various screening strategies for a variety of cancers. Specifically, in regard to PSA screening, they ranked it what they termed a "Level D", stating "**The USPSTF recommends against screening for prostate cancer**. The USPSTF concludes that the current evidence is insufficient to assess the balance of benefits and harms of prostate cancer screening"   Four years later, in 2012, they amended their recommendation to a Level C for men under 70, recommending physicians "selectively offering or providing this service to individual patients based on professional judgment and patient preferences. There is at lest moderate certainty that the net benefit is small." In 2018, the USPTF recommendation for men age 55-69 is still level C, and for men over 70, "The USPSTF recommends against PSA-based screening for prostate cancer in men 70 years and older." - Level D.

Why such reluctance to recommend an inexpensive blood test? The USPTF recommendations (2008 and 2012) were based on a review of three studies involving a combined total of 237,000 men. The USPTF panel is made up of physicians and statisticians who analyzed the data and concluded that PSA is an inadequate indicator of cancer, did not reduce mortality from prostate cancer, and too often led to a trans-rectal ultrasound biopsies that found cancer in "only" 25-30% of those who underwent the procedure. Side effects of transrectal ultrasounds and biopsies include blood in the urine, infection, urinary retention, and rarely sepsis. If you've read the last couple of chapters, I'm sure you can understand how unpleasant and concerning some of these side effects can be, and I can attest that these unpleasant side effects do happen, a topic I'll address further on. But let's get back to the USPTF recommendation.

I attended the 2008 annual American Urologic Association meeting where the USPTF first announced its recommendations. I found it interesting that these recommendations would be presented at a conference of urologists, given that not a single urologist or oncologist (cancer expert) was among the committee members who had "analyzed the 3 studies. Instead, the committee studying the impact PSA had on prostate cancer survival was made up of family practice, internal medicine and pediatric physicians, as well as statisticians. Not to denigrate these specialties, but when it comes to evaluating prostate health, it's urologists you turn to. Thus, it was no surprise when the panel moderator asked a room of nearly 1,000 urologists, "Does anyone in this room agree with this recommendation?" not a single person in the room raised their hand. What's more, the presentations that followed included a variety of presentations from statisticians, urologists, and oncologists who were not part of the USPTF committee (including the *authors of the three studies* the USPTF based their findings on) and explained, with data and evidence, why their "Level D" ranking of no net benefit was wrong and potentially dangerous.

So why did the USPTF make that recommendation? For starters, the panelists lumped all men 55 and over in one group. In other words they did not stratify for age. The problem with this is that a 75 year old is likely not to benefit from screening, whereas a 55 year old who may benefit, in terms of survival.

They concluded that the test was "too sensitive," or "positive too often" and thus detected small, slow-growing cancers that may not need to be treated at all, because the man would likely die from something else before the cancer got him. So it may be true that early detection of a small localized prostate cancer is likely not going to cause problems for a 75 year old. On the other hand, early detection and treatment of a localized cancer in a 55 year old is potentially life saving. This may be oversimplification of a complicated problem, but the bottom line is that by lumping 50 year olds with 70 year old men, the USPTF did not take into account the differences in risk of having a significant life threatening cancer these men of different ages faced.

The USPTF panel also found the test lacked "specificity," meaning there were too many "false positives" (a PSA greater than 4, and biopsy negative is a "false positive"), which could lead to unnecessary, invasive or expensive tests. A false positive—telling someone they may have cancer when they don't—can also cause undo anxiety. No one wants to undergo a biopsy and risk infection, much less the discomfort of the procedure, due to a PSA greater than 4 when a cancer is not detected (a false positive). On the other hand, a potential concern would be false negatives (a PSA < 4 when cancer is present), resulting in a false sense of security when there really is cancer. We'd much rather work with a test that has too many false positives, than one with too many false negatives. Fortunately, false negatives, a report of "normal levels" (even though I will repeat that there is no such thing as a "normal PSA") occur in fewer than 10% of men with clinically significant prostate cancer. And many of those men with a "normal" PSA but clinically significant prostate cancer, will have an abnormal prostate exam, and could also have an abnormal MRI. In other words, their cancer is likely to be caught.

We'll get back to the USPTF in a minute, but for now, rather than talk about PSA in terms of positive, negative, high, low, specificity, and sensitivity. However, I'd like to think about it in a different way. As I've suggested, *there is no such thing as a high or low PSA, and there is no such thing as a "normal" or "abnormal" PSA*. Think of it this way. Every man has a unique PSA and a unique risk of having prostate cancer. Taking it a step further, every prostate cancer risk can be viewed as the overall risk of any prostate cancer, and the risk of having clinically significant prostate cancer, the kind that can grow fast, spread to bones, lymph nodes and beyond, and may take your life.

There are several variables that affect the PSA result, including age, size of the prostate, presence or absence of inflammation in the prostate, and others. Here's what you want to keep in mind.

- **PSA goes up as men get older.** PSA goes up with each decade, so a PSA of 4 in a 50 year old is associated with a much higher risk of significant cancer than a PSA of 4 in a 70 year old man.

- **PSA goes up as the prostate enlarges.** Most urologists have an ultrasound machine in their offices to accurately measure the volume of the prostate, which takes less than three minutes to accurately measure. A smaller prostate would be expected to have a lower PSA than a larger one.

- **Infections or inflammation will elevate the PSA.** Infections of any type that affect the urinary tract, prostate, bladder, even an infection originating in the kidney can cause a high PSA. It's recently been discovered that a Covid 19 infection will cause the PSA to go up, which implies that during a Covid infection, the virus hit the prostate. https://www.ncbi.nlm.nih.gov/pmc/articles/PMC8493783/

- **Ejaculation will cause PSA to go up.** When I would get a referral for a man with an elevated PSA, one of the first questions I would ask would be, "Do you remember if you'd had sex before you got the blood drawn?" If they answered that they had sex that morning or even the night before, I'd schedule a repeat PSA test, and ask them to refrain from sex three days prior to the blood draw. It was common to see the PSA level drop in those cases.

- **A catheter or biopsy of the prostate will make PSA go up.** Minimally invasive procedures such as biopsies of the prostate or draining the urinary tract through a catheter or other instrument will elevate PSA levels.

- **Certain drugs will lower PSA.** The most common class of drugs that lower PSA are drugs that are used to treat prostate cancer. Hormone ablation therapy (drugs like Lupron) and chemotherapy (Taxotere) will lower PSA to undetectable levels (<0.05). That's how we know if the therapy is working (discussed in detail in the next chapter on prostate cancer). Drugs to treat benign enlargement of the prostate (such as Proscar/finasteride and Avodart/dutasteride), as well as to treat hair loss, are enzyme inhibitors which can lower PSA. NSAIDs (non-steroidal anti-inflammatory drugs like Advil or Motrin), statins (to lower cholesterol) and thiazide diuretics (used to tread edema, congestive heart failure and high blood pressure) also lower PSA. Your urologist should take into consideration that if you are taking any of these drugs, you will have a lower PSA that could underestimate your risk of cancer.
- **Prostate massage elevates PSA.** A digital rectal exam will not affect your PSA, but an aggressive prostate massage used to diagnose prostatitis does. So if you go to your doctor with vague symptoms of prostatitis, and s/he does a rectal exam of your prostate with massage, and then sends you to the lab for a PSA, that PSA is going to be higher than if the PSA were done prior to the exam/massage.

As these variables show, the risk of cancer can't be evaluated just by looking at a number measuring your PSA. It's important to consider multiple factors. I favor thinking of PSA as representing a unique value for a given man at a point in time, and that the PSA value for that man is associated with his risk of having prostate cancer. Your

PSA is just one variable—albeit an important value—that we consider along with each man's other variables, such as age, co-existing health problems, and medications, in assessing whether he should have more invasive diagnostic tests to determine or rule out if he has prostate cancer. We call this risk assessment.

PSA and Risk Assessment

Because PSA is an early detection tool and won't diagnose cancer, it's important to understand its limitations and its value in assessing risk. So instead of looking at PSA as positive or negative, high or low, let's look at it in terms of individual risk assessment. Then we can have a shared decision making conversation about further tests and procedures.

If you want to know what your individual risk is of having clinically significant prostate cancer (the kind that spreads or kills people) you need to have a PSA. A rectal exam can also help with risk assessment, preferably performed by a doctor who is skilled at detecting nodules and abnormalities. If you see a urologist, he/she will always do a rectal exam to feel your prostate. I still recommend that primary care providers do rectal exams. It takes less than 30 seconds, a glove that costs less than a nickel, and some lube. The reason for this is because there are still some men who will have hard abnormal prostates and low risk PSA values. Moreover, a simple rectal test can determine if there are any rectal anomalies or rectal cancer. Once you have your PSA level and a rectal exam, you or your doctor can go online and Google, "Prostate cancer risk calculator."

Here's how the risk calculators work: You and/or your doctor plugs in a set of variables such as age, PSA, rectal exam, family history, race, history of prior biopsy, and more depending on the calculator. Based on the variables, you will get an analysis of what your overall risk is of having prostate cancer, what your risk is of not having cancer, and what your risk is of having "clinically significant" cancers. If your risk that you can tolerate for having clinically *insignificant* prostate cancer is low, then you may choose not to have a biopsy. But, you do want to keep an eye on your PSA over time to see if there are any significant changes—it's in those changes that our concern rises or falls. And again, there are many variables to take into consideration that might affect those changes, such as your increasing age, the size of your prostate, any medications you've started or stopped taking, that sort of thing. Here's an example of a risk calculator that I like - http://www.clevelandclinic.org/lp/prostate-cancer-risk-assessment/

The USPTF didn't factor in these variables in making their recommendation. Instead, they treated every man's PSA as the sole variable to consider. The problem with the three studies the USPTF evaluated is that the USPTF committee of non-urologists and non-oncologists misinterpreted the studies and came to erroneous conclusions. It's important that I explain further.

When studies are designed to test whether screening a population will benefit a population (in this case men between the ages of 55 and 75), we divide the population into two groups - a group to be screened and a control group. The men in the screened group would be tested (PSA), diagnosed (ultrasound guided biopsy), and then treated. The control group would not be tested until there was reason to test (symptoms) and then diagnosed if the symptoms warranted a biopsy, and then treated. In these studies, men in each group were followed to see if and when they died from prostate cancer. Unfortunately, all three studies are significantly flawed.

The methods by which both groups were "screened" or "not screened" were variable. Many men in the control group had their PSAs checked, which means the control group was contaminated. There was variability in both groups as to how often PSAs were checked. There was variability in both groups in terms of how the biopsies were done (for example, how many cores of tissue were obtained and from what part of the prostate), the timing of the biopsies, and whether or not repeat biopsies were done if the first one came back negative and the PSA was still "abnormal".

When cancer was diagnosed, the treatment of men with cancer in both groups (screened and control) received was extremely variable, but these variables weren't factored in when the two groups were compared.. As I said above, in each of the three studies upon which the USPTF based their flawed recommendation, the"control group" included participants who had had PSA tests and who were then treated for prostate cancer. With all that in mind, of course you are not going to be able to tell the difference between the control and screened groups. For an accurate assessment of the impact of PSA, the control group should not have been tested with PSA, and only treated for prostate cancer after presenting with symptoms (something I've already told you is *rare when the cancer is still localized and treatable.*

Furthermore, in all three studies the USPTF evaluated, there was no separation into different groups according to age, medical co-morbidities (other illnesses or disorders), or the grade or stage of any cancer detected. In other words, everybody was lumped in with everyone else. Think about it—if you had two groups of men and wanted to determine who might live longer from early cancer detection, a healthy 50 year old man or a 75 year old man with diabetes, hypertension and heart disease, who is likely to benefit? Clearly, the healthy 50 year old. Likewise, a man with intermediate grade cancer confined to the prostate is more likely to benefit than one who has high grade metastatic cancer that has already spread to his lymph nodes. But these diverse men were all lumped together in the studies, making it impossible to accurately assess the benefits of PSA.

Now let's return to the problem of a high false positive rate. The USPTF argued that a trans-rectal ultrasound and biopsy of the prostate is positive for cancer "only 25 to 33%" of the time. They argued that three quarters of men with high PSA levels are put through an invasive procedure that can have significant complications including hematuria, infection, urinary retention, and even sepsis. I've personally seen all these complications, though infrequently (less than 2%) so I won't argue that they aren't a problem. But in most cases these issues are self-limiting—meaning they resolve on their own and are to be expected. In all the biopsies I've done over the course of my 35 year career, I can think of only having to stop the bleeding with a small suture less than five times. As for infections, these can be avoided with a proper course of antibiotics. Sepsis usually occurs if the patient has been on antibiotics recently and has developed a resistance to that particular antibiotic. Most urologists are aware of this issue and will choose an intramuscular or intravenous antibiotic to avoid sepsis. The overall complication rate from trans-rectal ultrasounds and biopsies was less than two percent of the prostate biopsies I conducted.

And yes, a biopsy can hurt if not done correctly. But, we routinely inject a local anesthetic around the nerves that go along the side of the prostate. With ultrasound, we can direct a needle with local anesthetic to the precise area we need to numb, so that there is minimal to no pain at all.

The conclusions of the USPTF were based on earlier technologies, and earlier experiences with PSA. The studies they evaluated were done at a time when most urologists were doing fewer biopsies, and no one routinely used local anesthesia to minimize or eliminate pain from the biopsy. It was also a time when few knew how to minimize the risk of infection. But things have changed a lot since then, and the risks are much less. What hasn't changed as much is the USPTF recommendations.

Their recommendation to avoid PSA screening made in 2008 led to a striking decrease in PSA screening. Between 2008 and 2018 there was a dramatic *increase* in the number of men initially diagnosed with advanced and metastatic disease. Following enormous criticism leveled at USPTF recommendation, in 2012 they amended their recommendation to suggest that for men between the ages of 55 and 69, it should be an individual decision based on "professional judgment" and "patient preferences," but for those who do not "express a preference" for "screening" (we're talking about a simple blood test and rectal exam), it should not be done. This change, from a Level D ranking to a Level C ranking, is simply not enough, in my opinion.

Still, consider just whose professional judgment they're talking about, and how patient preferences are shaped. I don't wish to denigrate primary care providers, such as family practice doctors or internal medicine physicians, because they provide excellent care and are in most cases on the frontlines of patient care. But the information they receive about prostate cancer, their training, and their experience with prostate cancer patients of all stages, is significantly different from that of a urologist or oncologist. When determining professional judgment, you want to listen to the advice of a specialist in urology and/or cancer when it comes to early detection for prostate cancer.

As for "patient preferences," consider what shapes your views of what you feel you need for your health and medical care. Patient preferences are shaped in part by a primary care doctor, but also by the media, the internet, and anecdotal experience. Ask yourself, is it better for my primary care doctor to determine if I should get a PSA, or for me to engage in a shared decision making conversation with my urologist, who can evaluate my PSA results along with other factors, to determine if I should have a biopsy (or more recently, an MRI, maybe even before the biopsy)? By understanding your individual risk of having aggressive prostate cancer, you want to know whether or not you have cancer. You may want to detect that cancer early, to avoid a great deal of morbidity from delayed diagnosis and even death. Another significant problem with the USPTF is that they only focus on mortality (death rate), yet completely ignore morbidity from advanced or metastatic cancer (more on this in a minute).

Let's think about late stage cancer, also known as advanced or metastatic cancer. When cancer is diagnosed, the USPTF criticizes the urologic community for diagnosing and treating too many indolent or slow-growing prostate cancers that may never harm a man. That concern may have been true in 2001, but by 2008, it was not the case, and is certainly not the case today. Most men with small volume (low stage), low grade (Gleason 6, which we'll discuss in the next chapter), are sometimes not treated, but rather watched closely, because 2/3 of these cancers will never cause problems in a man's life. This is called "active surveillance and is something we discuss in more detail in the next chapter. Prostate cancer can be a slow growing cancer, but for one third of those who have a so-called "slow growing" or "indolent" cancer, it can progress to something that is more aggressive and dangerous.

PSA velocity is another helpful measure in understanding the overall risk of having prostate cancer and may provide a clue to whether the cancer is low or high risk. PSA changes over time. The rate of change of PSA is called velocity. PSA doubling time is a variation of this idea and it is simply how long it takes for the PSA to double. If you've been diagnosed with prostate cancer, the longer the doubling time, the less risk of significant fast-growing cancer, the shorter the doubling time, the higher the risk. A PSA doubling time of less than a year in the absence of other factors that cause a rise in PSA is significant and should raise a red flag that something serious could be happening, regardless of whether you've been diagnosed with prostate cancer or not.

Since the Level D recommendation was made in 2008, we've seen a dramatic doubling of the incidence of advanced metastatic disease. Now over 20% of men diagnosed with prostate cancer will need to be on hormone ablation for the rest of their lives. Between 1990 and 2008 it was less than 10%. The side effects of hormone ablation include weakness, hot flashes, sweats, depression, breast enlargement, loss of libido, and impotence, to name a few. And once the cancer reaches the bones, the bones can become so weak they break easily and spontaneously. Cancer in the bones of the spine can lead to paralysis from compression of the spinal cord. Clearly, catching cancer before it reaches this stage is well worth the minor inconvenience of monitoring PSA—which at the time of this writing, is a simple $8 blood test in our lab at Kaiser in Portland.

So what about men younger than 55 or older than 69? If you fall into one of these categories, should you follow the USPTF guidelines and not get it? In my opinion, the most effective early detection program should start when men are in their forties. We know for a fact that men in their 40s who have a PSA of 1.5 or more have a greater than 50% chance of developing clinically significant prostate cancer during their life time. Those are the men who should be screened.

As for older men, I think that denying a healthy 75 year old man a PSA who is likely to live to age 85 or 90 is wrong. Why shouldn't his risk of cancer be taken as seriously as that of a younger man, if the cancer is potentially aggressive?

It's fine to talk about the benefits and harms of screening (I prefer to use the word "testing" rather than "screening" with your PCP, but what harm can come from an inexpensive blood test? Shouldn't you be able to weigh the risks of having a clinically-significant cancer against the minor risk of having a biopsy? The earlier you are diagnosed, the better your chance of being cured, and the sooner you are diagnosed, the better chance you have of never having metastatic prostate cancer, and never having to be on hormone therapy.

Despite these facts, the USPTF *did not even consider the benefit of PSA testing* preventing metastatic cancer! They only looked at death rates, and they did so with populations that were by definition problematic because they were not adequately distinguished by age, morbidity, or other variables. Considering how morbid and damaging (not to mention expensive) advanced and metastatic prostate cancer is, this is a terrible omission by the USPTF.

The bottom line is good, cost-effective early detection will lower the death rate and morbidity from cancer. One goal is to diagnose a cancer early, treat it when it's localized, and thus avoid a premature death from cancer. If the cancer is diagnosed when it's confined to the prostate (Stage 1 or 2), surviving five years after treatment without any evidence of cancer is 98%, at 10 years it is 96%, and 15 years 94%.

Another goal of appropriate PSA testing is to detect and treat early to avoid and prevent metastases and all of the morbidity associated with distant spread of disease. The 5-year survival if you have meta-static (typically cancer in bones or lymph nodes) or locally advanced disease (a large amount of cancer outside the prostate in the pelvis) is 30%. A good early detection program should be practical, cost-effec-tive tests should be non-invasive or minimally invasive, and there should be a high degree of sensitivity (few false negatives) and speci-ficity (few false positives).

Prior to PSA, over 50% of men had metastatic disease when they were first diagnosed. After PSA started being used more widely, we saw a dramatic reduction in the number of men who presented with metastatic disease to about 10%. That bears repeating—the incidence of metastatic or advanced disease decreased from 50% to 10% only 10 years after PSA was introduced into clinical practice. It rose only after the USTPF report advised against its use.

PSA is not a perfect screening test, mainly because it does not have high specificity, in other words, there are too many false positives. Still, as Dr. William Catalona says, "I believe that PSA-based testing (including PHI- Prostate Health Index) is the *best cancer blood test in all branches of medicine*, and certainly the best test currently available for early prostate cancer detection." https://www.urolo-gytimes.com/view/prostate-specific-antigen-based-screening-ush-ers-in-an-era-of-change

As Dr Catalona and others have said, PSA is not a perfect test. It's not specific enough (too many false positives) and doesn't correlate completely with which man has clinically significant prostate cancer and which man has indolent, slow growing, or clinically insignificant prostate cancer. Until recently, that distinction required a biopsy. However, the development of the multi-detector MRI has been a game changer. In fact, some early detection algorithms (particularly in Europe and other parts of the world), recommend a mpMRI *prior* to biopsy. If the MRI is normal, a biopsy is not done, and the PSA can be followed. In cases in which the PSA rises (high PSA velocity) the MRI can be repeated. If the MRI shows something, a more accurate or guided biopsy can be done. In the U.S., a man will sometimes be seen by a urologist for a "high PSA" and the biopsy comes back negative. Does that mean the urologist missed the cancer or is there no cancer? An MRI can help answer the question. A negative MRI after a negative biopsy can obviate the need for a second, third, or fourth biopsy.

There are other ways of making PSA more specific, and new technologies for improving risk assessment are continually being developed and put into use. Some of these tests have been around for over 30 years, and some are still being developed. They include testing for the percentage of free PSA, PSA density, PCA3 (this is a urine test), and isoPSA. These tests all represent an evolution in the early detection of prostate cancer. The goal is to diagnose clinically significant cancers in those men who will benefit from treatment, those men who can be cured, and those men who you would like not to suffer from metastatic disease. While at the same time, the tests do nor find clinically slow growing, small, indolent cancers that will never cause harm and do not need to be treated. These are things you will want to talk to your urologist about *before* you submit to a biopsy or repeat biopsy.

Caption: Risk Assessment Tools prior to biopsy or repeat biopsy. Note, this table is does not list all of the currently useful tests available. Some of these tests, particularly when combined, are sensitive in predicting the risk of high grade clinically significant potentially dangerous and lethal prostate cancer vs indolent and likely harmless cancer.

Age	Select MDX (urine)
Race	Rectal Exam
PSA	IsoPSA
Family History	Prior Biopsy
% Free PSA	genetic markers
PSA density	Stockholm - 3 (STHLM3)
PSA transition zone density	TMPRSS2:erg fusion
PSA velocity	Polygenic Risk Scores
PCA 3 (urine)	mpMRI
EPI prostate cancer (urine)	

Table 1. Prostate Cancer Risk Factor Variables

These are the references that I am citing with respect to the newer ways of increasing PSA specificity (fewer false positives, fewer unwarranted biopsies)

https://pubmed.ncbi.nlm.nih.gov/35969726/ (EPI test)

https://pubmed.ncbi.nlm.nih.gov/33941866/ (Select MDX)

both are urine tests

Stockholm 3 https://pubmed.ncbi.nlm.nih.gov/29331214/

IsoPSA https://pubmed.ncbi.nlm.nih.gov/30810464/ (I actually met with Arnon Chait from the Cleveland Clinic 10 years ago and my ex-partners participated in the clinical trials after I retired).

So if you've had any doubts about getting your PSA checked, rest assured that doing so will provide you with the data you and your physician need to keep you healthy. My hope is that no one reading this book dies from prostate cancer, so I will leave you with one final story. Back in the mid-1990s, I was talking with one of our residents who had recently admitted a man he diagnosed with a PSA of 600 and widespread bone metastasis. I asked if he'd ever had a PSA before his admission.

"No, never," the resident said.

"Is he insured?"

"Yes, he's been insured for twenty years."

"Had he seen a family doctor or internist over the past ten years?"

"Yes, many times."

That conversation got us to wondering—how many other men had we been treating for advanced cancer hadn't had their PSAs evaluated before their cancer had metastasized?

We started reviewing charts and found 100 men who came to us with undiagnosed high PSAs and metastatic cancer. Of those men, 85 of 100 had been insured. We looked at those 85 men to see if they had seen a primary care provider or a urologist during the decade before their diagnosis—all 85 had seen their PCP, none had seen a urologist. But why would they, since most prostate cancers are asymptomatic until they become advanced or metastatic?

We then dug deeper into their charts and asked how many of the 85 had either had a rectal exam, a PSA, or even a discussion about the risks and benefits of getting a PSA. *Of the 85 men with high PSAs and metastatic cancer, not a single one had had a PSA or rectal exam! And we saw no evidence that there had even been a discussion of having one!*

We can only speculate as to how many of these men might never have developed such devastating disease had their PSAs been evaluated early on and their cancer detected before it had metastasized.

Conclusion

Now that you are armed with the information, I hope you will include a PSA blood test in your preventive health care and engage in shared decision making discussions with your doctor about the result of the test. Please don't be alarmed if your PSA is not "normal" because now you know that there is no such thing. Again, your PSA is one variable among several that predict your risk of having prostate cancer. Chances are a "high" or "abnormal" PSA may not be due to cancer, but if it is cancer, you're more likely to survive or not have to suffer from metastasis or the treatment of metastases if you are diagnosed with cancer early. If it is cancer, you'll want to read the next chapter, to learn what that means and how to beat it.

PSA FOR PRIMARY CARE CLINICIANS

"Should I get a PSA?"

It depends. Who is asking, and why?

If the question is being asked by a 45-year-old man, the answer is going to be different than if it's being asked by 75 year old. If you are a primary care clinician, you may confused about current recommendations regarding screening for prostate cancer. The answer is complicated and fraught with bias. You've been told one thing by the USPTF and your medical societies to "leave it up to the patient", and another thing by your urology colleagues. Unfortunately, the controversy over PSA screening for prostate cancer is still with us after 40 years of experience.

I practiced urology for 35 years. I started my residency in urology at Oregon Health Science University in 1979, eight to 10 years before urologists began using PSA.

I have witnessed the evolution of prostate cancer "screening" using PSA. I was there before the controversy started, and I'm still here in the middle of the fight. The "fight?" Yes, the fight. In one corner are the doubters, the "non-screeners," physicians who take their cues from the US Preventative Task force 2012 level D (since revised to Level C in 2018) - "we don't need to screen for prostate cancer by doing PSAs on our patients because most prostate cancers are indolent and slow growing and men aren't going to die from prostate cancer. The treatment (surgery, radiation, hormones) is worse than the disease."

In the other corner are urologists, oncologists, and radiation oncologists who believe that early detection of prostate cancer using PSA as an initial marker is not only possible, but in fact saves lives. More importantly early detection prevents morbidity from advanced and/or metastatic disease.

In 1980 PSA was still in research labs. By mid-80s doctors realized that PSA was a more sensitive test for detecting prostate cancer. Acid phosphatase (blood test), was elevated in advanced/metastatic prostate cancer, but not as sensitive for prostate cancer as PSA. Prior to PSA, the only way to detect localized prostate cancer was by digital rectal exam (DRE), by investigating symptoms of bladder outlet obstruction, or investigating symptoms of advanced/metastatic disease.

Before the mid-80s, if a nodule was felt, a blind biopsy using only finger guidance was done. A positive biopsy, normal acid phos, negative bone and CT scan meant "localized prostate cancer." That patient was offered surgery (usually a radical retro-pubic prostatectomy) or external beam radiation therapy. This was rare. From 1979 to 1982 I scrubbed on two radical prostatectomies. After PSA had been around for 15 years, I was doing two radical prostatectomies a week, roughly 100 a year.

Half the prostate cancer patients in the early 80s had advanced or metastatic disease. If the patient had locally advanced disease, but no metastases (Stage 'C'), he would be treated with radiation. 25% of patients were found to have prostate cancer after a TURP, stage A1 (fewer than 5% of chips +) or A2 (greater than 5% of chips +). At the Portland VA typically half of our patients on the ward were being treated for metastatic prostate cancer with IV stilphosterol and/or radiation therapy to distant mets, or painful bone mets in danger of pathologic fracture.

What happened over the next four decades with respect to PSA in the US (things are different in other countries) is both phenomenal and tragic. With millions of PSAs and prostate biopsies being done, the incidence of prostate cancer increased, however the percent of patients presenting with advanced and metastatic disease fell from 50% to less than 10%. Mortality from prostate cancer declined.

We learned that PSA was an excellent test to assess response to treatment. An undetectable PSA after treatment was indicative of an excellent response to treatment (surgery, radiation, even hormone ablation for treatment of metastatic disease). A rising PSA after treatment was indicative of recurrence.

We learned about PSA velocity (change in PSA over time), PSA density (PSA/prostate volume), % free PSA, PCA3 (prostate cancer antigen urine test), isoPSA, and recently newer tests like ExoDx (urine biomarker). All of these variations and tests have been helpful in refining the sensitivity and specificity of PSA based screening. Add to those tools multi-parametric MRI.

Prostate cancer incidence increases 10% each decade. A 50-year-old man has a 50% chance of having "prostate cancer" in his prostate, a 60 year old, 60%, etc. Obviously, not all prostate cancers are "clinically significant," meaning they are slow growing, indolent, and will never cause any problem for the duration of that man's life, which is why many doctors will tell patients "You are more likely to die *with* prostate cancer than *from* prostate cancer."

This created problems because many clinically insignificant cancers were unnecessarily treated. With over treatment came significant complications - impotence, incontinence, and post surgical and radiation complications.

The USPTF issued a Level D recommendation against PSA-based screening (2008 and 2012). The recommendation was based on 3 studies (PLOC, ERSPC, and Gothenburg). All three studies are all flawed for a variety of reasons, and misinterpreted by the USPFT. Not one urologist or oncologist was on the USPTF committee. The USPFT recommendation has been extensively criticized in the literature. Morbidity from metastatic disease and treatment is not a part of their analysis. Nor were technological advances (laparoscopic robotic assisted prostatectomy particularly) considered. As a result of the flawed recommendation by the USPTF, there was an increase in advanced/metastatic disease, which prompted revision of their recommendation to Level C in 2018.

Today the two camps are still far apart on early detection of prostate cancer. Like other conflicting beliefs in 2023, this conflict makes no sense and doesn't have to be. Thousands of men are still presenting with advanced and metastatic prostate cancer. It is estimated that 35,000 men will die of prostate cancer in 2023. Hundreds of thousands more will require treatment of metastatic disease.

"Who are these men? Have they ever had a PSA or digital rectal exam?" In the mid 90s we reviewed 100 consecutive patients who presented with advanced or metastatic prostate cancer. Many had PSAs over 100. We asked "how many had heath care insurance during the 10 years prior to presentation?" 85. We then wondered "How many had a PSA and/or a DRE within 10 years of being diagnosed with metastatic/advanced disease?" Zero! (0!). And, "How many had a documented 'shared decision making' conversations regarding the "potential harms/risks vs benefits" of getting a PSA?" Again, zero.

The April 2023 AUA Guideline *Early Detection of Prostate Cancer: AUA/SUO Guideline (2023)* states "Clinicians should engage in shared decision-making (SDM) with people for whom prostate cancer screening would be appropriate and proceed based on a person's values and preferences. (*Clinical Principle*)" https://www.auanet.org/guidelines-and-quality/guidelines/early-detection-of-prostate-cancer-guidelines. From the May 2018 USPTF recommendation - "Based on a review of the evidence, the Task Force recommends that men aged 55 to 69 years **make an individual decision** about whether to be screened after a conversation with their clinician about the potential benefits and harms. For men 70 years and older, the potential benefits do not outweigh the expected harms, and these men should not be routinely screened for prostate cancer." https://www.uspreventiveservicestaskforce.org/uspstf/announcements/final-recommendation-statement-screening-prostate-cancer#:~:text=Based%20on%20a%20review%20of,the%20potential%20benefits%20and%20harms.

Most clinicians do not have the time to do a robust, factual, non-biased "shared decision making" conversation. And, it's not the patient's responsibility to be informed enough to be able to have a conversation about whether or not to have a PSA.

The disconnect between primary care and urology need not exist. Urologists are not interested in doing biopsies on a patients with PSAs (and other indicators - MRI Pi-RAD of 3-5, ExoDx > 15, and more) indicative of low risk indolent prostate cancer. Urologists are not interested in treating cancers that don't need treatment. In fact, a full third of patients who have positive biopsies are offered active surveillance. Likewise, primary care physicians are not interested in doing lots of PSAs, which leads to unnecessary biopsies and unnecessary treatment causing impotence, incontinence, and worse, only to benefit a small number of those men. And, with the advent of mp-MRI, some men referred to a urologist for an "elevated PSA" may elect active surveillance without a biopsy if the MRI is negative (Pi-Rad 1 or 2).

We know enough about PSA (and DRE) to be able to inform a man of his risk of having a ***clinically significant*** versus ***indolent*** CaP PRIOR to TRUS/bx. Risk calculators are readily available and a man can then decide, based upon his risk, whether or not to have a biopsy.

If the biopsy is positive, urologists have the necessary information to have a robust SDM conversation about whether or NOT treatment is indicated, based on individual preferences, and what each treatment (potential harms, risks, benefits) entails.

For four decades urologists have improved the specificity of PSA as an initial early detection tool. The days of a normal PSA being < 4 have long passed. Every man has an individual risk of developing clinically significant and potentially dangerous prostate cancer based on tons of good studies and evidence (mpMRI, enhanced PSA interpretation using %freePSA, PSA density, PSA velocity, isoPSA, urine biomarkers (PCA3, ExoDx), genetic markers, and more!

If you and your patient want to know the risk of having a clinically significant prostate cancer, please just get the PSA, and then find someone who can have an informed shared decision making conversation about what to do next.

CHAPTER 7

Prostate Cancer[vii]

As the last chapter showed, it wasn't that long ago that a diagnosis of prostate cancer was a devastating diagnosis, due primarily to the lack of symptoms until the disease had metastasized beyond the prostate. Many men who were diagnosed with prostate cancer would die within a few years, if not sooner. PSA has been around for over 35 years, and urologists have become very good at using PSA as a tool for early diagnosis of prostate cancer in those men who would benefit the most. Along with better diagnostic tests (especially MRI), most men who are diagnosed early today can be cured, or at the very least, their cancer will be managed into their old age. Unfortunately, with our remarkable progress in diagnosing and treating prostate cancer, there is the perception among many that no one dies from prostate cancer anymore. That perception is not always the case. Indeed, the myth that "no one dies from prostate cancer" is wrong, if not absurd - 31,636 men died of prostate cancer in 2021 in the US[viii].

The truth is, prostate cancer is nothing to ignore. One out of nine men will be diagnosed with prostate cancer during their lifetime, making it the second most common cancer in men in the United States (after skin cancer) with over 200,000 new cases of prostate cancer each year, The death rate is still significant. Many of these deaths can be prevented if the cancer is caught early. As I showed in the last chapter, many primary care doctors still follow the USPTF (US Preventative Task Force) guideline that discourages "PSA screening."

What do you need to know if you get diagnosed with prostate cancer? You need to know your treatment options, as well as some basic facts about this potentially devastating, but often curable, disease. If you are properly informed you'll be better able to make a decision about whether or not to be treated. If you do decide to be treated, the treatment should be tailored to your goals,lifestyle, and values. You are entitled to know how you will benefit from whatever treatment you choose, and what risks you'll be taking.

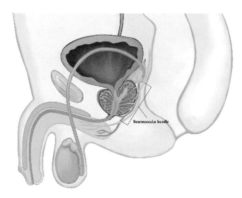

Nerves for erection can be spared in "nerve sparing" prostatectomy on one or both sides in some cases, enhancing chances of normal sexual function after surgery. The nerves may not be spared in some cases if the cancer is close to the nerves. In those cases, it's advised to remove the nerves to get all of the cancer out. As you'll see on the chapter on erectile dysfunction, there are several ways of treating ED if the neuromuscular bundle has been removed.

There are some prostate cancers that are slow-growing and may take years to spread beyond the prostate, if ever. There are other prostate cancers that are fast growing and are more likely to spread (metastasize). Even the most aggressive forms (we call these "clinically significant") can usually be cured if caught early. Understanding how prostate cancer grows and the factors that influence that growth will help you to understand your diagnosis and options for treatment. At the beginning of this discussion, it's useful to understand how we "grade" and "stage" cancer, which helps to understand potential treatment options.

Cancer Grade and Gleason Score

Prostate cancer is the abnormal growth of the glands in the prostate. When we examine the glands under a microscope, we look at the pattern of these glands and the cells that comprise them to determine their "grade." This grade corresponds to a number, 1-5, and is what is termed the "Gleason Grade." The "Gleason Scoring System," is named after the pathologist Donald Gleason who in 1966 developed a way to evaluate cancer cell proliferation.

We evaluate the possibility of you having prostate cancer by taking multiple biopsies (usually twelve, but this can vary) from different locations in the prostate to see if cancer is present. If the pathologist sees prostate cancer in any or all of the cores, she will determine how much of that core has cancer in it. Then, based on the appearance of the cells and how they are arranged, the pathologist will assign as Gleason Grade to each cancer. If the cells and arrangement of the glands indicate a slow-growing cancer, the Gleason Grade is lower. This type of cancer is described as "well differentiated." The more abnormal the cells and arrangement of the glands are, the higher the Gleason grade. We call this type of cancer "poorly differentiated." So a Gleason grade of 5 implies that the cancer is fast growing and potentially fatal, whereas a 1 would be considered slow-growing and potentially curable.

Generally speaking, low volume (meaning only a few of the cores have cancer, and the amount of cancer in each core is small), well differentiated cancers are slow growing, indolent, and not clinically significant, whereas intermediate and poorly differentiated cancers *are* clinically significant. There can be different cancer grades in each of the samples, or there can be just one grade (again, a Gleason Grade number ranges from 1-5). The Primary Grade is the most common grade seen in each of the samples. The Secondary Grade represents the second most common grade noted. The *Gleason Score* is the sum of the primary Gleason grade added to the Secondary grade. For example, if you have a Gleason Grade of 3 for your primary grade, and 4 for your secondary grade, you have a Gleason Score of 7 (3 + 4 = 7).

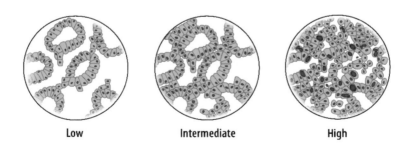

| Low | Intermediate | High |

Grades of Adenocarcinoma of the Prostate

Depending on the how much cancer is seen in each of the specimens, a Gleason score of 6 or under is considered slow growing or "clinically insignificant. The higher the score, the greater the risk of a fast growing cancer, one that may spread to other organs (usually lymph nodes or bones).

GLEASON SCORE

$\leq$ 6 Unlikely to grow or spread

  7 May grow or spread

$\geq$ 8 Likely to grow or spread

There's more to risk than just the Gleason Score. When we talk about "risk" in cancer, we're talking about the risk of the cancer spreading beyond the prostate and into the bones, bloodstream and/or lymph nodes, as well as other tissues and organs. Ultimately, the greatest risk is death. Given this definition of risk, we want to be sure we're evaluating each patient's risk as comprehensively as possible. That's where the PSA and imaging like MRI (Magnetic Resonance Imaging) are useful. Recall from the last chapter that we assess risk using PSA. When a cancer is diagnosed. The higher the PSA in a person with known cancer, the greater the risk of that cancer behaving badly.

Another way of evaluating risk in addition to the Gleason Score and PSA is the stage of the tumor, or T-stage. If cancer is found in your prostate, we evaluate it by what we call the TNM system. T represents the Tumor itself—how big it is, where it is located (for example, if it is palpable and felt on a digital rectal exam, or if it is found in the seminal vesicles or has spread into the bladder. N represents

Nodes —usually the first place prostate cancer spreads is to the pelvic lymph nodes, but as the spread progresses, other lymph nodes outside the pelvis may be involved. M represents Metastasis—when the cancer has spread to places other than lymph nodes, usually bones, but can also be seen in liver, lungs, and other organs or tissues.

The following chart will give you an idea of how tumor stage is ranked:

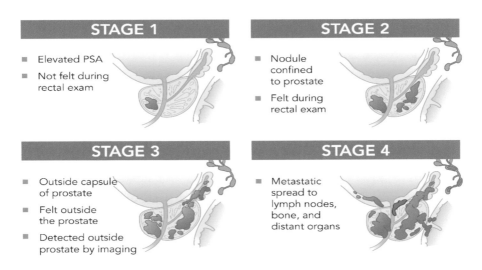

Stages of Prostate Cancer (start at top left – A, top right B, low left C, low right D

Based on your PSA and Gleason Score results from your biopsy, your urologist will assess whether or not you have a clinically signifi-cant (potentially dangerous) or clinically insignificant cancer (indo-lent, usually small volume, Gleason Score of 6 or less). If you have a clinically significant cancer, your urologist will order an MRI or CT of the pelvis and abdomen, and a bone scan to further stage your can-cer. Depending on the TNM stage and the Gleason Score, you are now ready to have a shared decision making discussion about what to do about your cancer. If you have a small amount of cancer with a Gleason Score of 6 or less, you will also have a discussion about no treatment, or active surveillance.

This discussion is important but can be complicated and confusing. Try to keep it simple by asking "if I have this treatment, what are my chances of being alive in 5, 10, and 15 years? What are my chances of being alive, but having to deal with this cancer again in 5, 10, and 15 years? What are the risks and benefits of the treatment you are proposing, compared to other treatments available? Are the complications permanent or can they be fixed?"

Your Treatment Options

Before discussing specific treatment options for your cancer, it's useful to understand how prostate cancer spreads. Prostate cancer feeds on hormones—specifically male hormone or testosterone. Testosterone is a type of hormone called an androgen, which is responsible for sperm production and male characteristics such as muscle mass, body hair growth, libido, erectile function and aggression. Testosterone is made in the testes (with a small amount made in the adrenal glands located just above the kidneys) and effects both benign and cancerous prostate tissue. When you have prostate cancer, cancer cells are stimulated to grow by testosterone and small amounts of other androgens causing the cells to proliferate. As they proliferate, they may eventually spread beyond the prostate to other tissues, most commonly lymph nodes, pelvic bones, spine, and ribs. Cancer cells can also be seen in the bloodstream. Cancer cells in the bloodstream may be deposited in other organs in the body like liver or lungs.

The goal of your shared making discussion should be to arrive at a course of treatment (or no treatment in the case of active surveillance) that best fits with your personal and unique concerns. It's all a matter of how much risk you are willing to accept from both the cancer and the treatment of your cancer.

There are five ways of "treating" your cancer. Sometimes a combination of treatments (for example, radiation and surgery, or hormone ablation and radiation) will produce a better outcome (survival with or without cancer and prevention of metastatic disease). These are your potential options[ix].

- Active surveillance
- Surgery
- Radiation
- Hormone Therapy
- Ablative Therapy (destroying the cancer cells)

Active Surveillance

Because most prostate cancer is slow-growing, if your life expectancy is less than ten years (based on your age and health status, including other diseases or disorders such as heart or lung disease or diabetes), you and your urologist may opt for Active Surveillance. You may be a good candidate for active surveillance is you have a low volume, Gleason Score of 6 cancer. Because some prostate cancers are slow growing, the reason not to treat is that the treatment may not lengthen your life, and the treatment itself may impede the quality of your life.

The decision to not treat and do AS depends on the TNM stage and the Gleason score. Various institutions have different recommendations for who qualifies for AS. In general, the T stage must be T1 or very low volume T2, and the Gleason score should be 6 or less. (Though there are some institutions that will offer AS to Gleason 3+4 patients).

Active Surveillance does not mean ignoring your cancer. If your physician tells you s/he "wants to keep an eye on it," what that might mean is either Active Surveillance or Watchful Waiting—waiting to see if other symptoms arise or the tumor becomes palpable. Watchful Waiting is common for elderly men or men with other medical problems who have low risk, slow-growing cancers. Why subject them to invasive treatments that could cause more problems than they already have, especially when treatment is unlikely to lengthen or improve the quality of their lives?

Active Surveillance is for younger generally healthy men. It means having regular PSA tests, usually every six months, along with further biopsies if the PSA changes, possibly every one to three years. Currently the use of MRI is becoming more important in diagnosing cancers that are being followed with active surveillance, while at the same time limiting the number of repeat biopsies. Some prostate cancers are T1 or small volume T2, with a Gleason score of 6. These cancers may not change over time, they are the clinically insignificant or indolent cancers discussed above. However, we do know that 30-35% of prostate cancers initially thought to be harmless indolent cancers will change and progress to a higher Gleason grade (4 or 5), or will grow and become a higher T stage (large T2 or T3). It's at this point that you, as well as other men who are not candidates for active surveillance will want to discuss treatment.

Surgery

Surgery for prostate cancer is called a radical prostatectomy. This means removal of the entire prostate, including the seminal vesicles (two small glands behind the prostate that join the vas deferens and empty semen and sperm into the prostate during ejaculation). In most cases, the surgeon will access the prostate through the abdominal wall behind the pubic bone, a procedure called "Retropubic." (In some cases, such as when the abdominal wall contains too much fat or the lymph nodes are involved, the prostate is accessed via the perineum, the space between the scrotum and rectum, but these days that procedure is extremely rare.)

In the past, prostatectomies were made with an incision from the belly button to the pubic bone, a method known as an Open Prostatectomy. That method is uncommon now, because we can perform the surgery using much smaller incisions through which "scopes" and interments are placed. This is called laparoscopy. There are two forms of laparoscopy used for prostatectomies, Robotic-Assisted Laparoscopic and Pure Laparoscopic (which means no robot is involved). Almost 90% of the prostatectomies performed in the United States today are Robotic-Assisted, using the da Vinci® System.

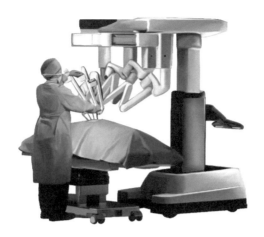

Robotic Assisted Laparoscopic Radical Prostatectomy

If in consultation with your healthcare team you opt for a Robotic-Assisted prostatectomy, your physician will arrange for you to have blood and urine tests beforehand, as well as an ECG—and electrocardiogram—to ensure your heart is in good working order. The night before the surgery, you will not be able to eat anything. You'll be put on a clear liquid diet the day before, and you'll have to drink a bottle of Magnesium Citrate to clear your bowels, just as if you were preparing for a routine colonoscopy. It will also be important to refrain from smoking cigarettes (including vaping) or taking aspirin, as both nicotine and aspirin can increase your blood loss. Although there is minimal bleeding with laparoscopy, anything that thins the blood can lead to problems.

On the morning of the surgery, you won't be able to drink anything unless your surgery is scheduled for late in the day, in which case you can have clear liquids in the morning. You may be given an epidural (an injection in your back numbing you from the waist down), prior to general anesthesia, or you might not, depending on the preference of your physician and anesthesiologist. Either way, you will be given a general anesthesia, so you won't be conscious for the surgery itself.

Two surgeons will perform the surgery, one to insert the laparoscopes and instruments and then attach them to the robotic arms, and another to control the robot from a console and perform the operation. Your abdominal cavity will be filled with carbon dioxide. Four to six small incisions will be made, each about one-half inch long, in an arc below your belly button. A camera and robotic instruments are then placed through these keyhole incisions or "ports," and then attached to the robot. The camera provides a magnified three-dimensional image of the abdominal cavity, enabling the surgeon to dissect the prostate and seminal vesicles free without ever putting his/her hands into the abdominal cavity.

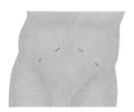 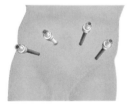

Port Placement for Laparoscopic Radical Prostatectomy

Depending on the tumor grade and stage, the surgeon may dissect the lymph nodes along the main blood vessels in the pelvis. The nerves responsible for erection are adherent to the prostate at 5 and 7 o'clock. Depending on the location of your cancer (how close it is to the nerves, and how close it is to the end of the prostate) the surgeon may elect to spare your nerves. This is called "nerve sparing" and will improve but not guarantee your chances of getting erections later. In some cases, depending on the tumor, nerve sparing on one or both sides might not be possible.

Once the prostate and any other affected tissues are removed through a small incision, the bladder is connected to the urethra. This is called an "anastomosis." The connection between the bladder and urethra is done over a catheter, which allows the connection to heal. The bladder end of the catheter is held in the bladder by a balloon filled with water about the size smaller than a golf ball. The catheter will drain urine from the bladder for 7-14 days (depending on surgeon preference). The small incisions are then closed. The entire procedure takes from 2 to 3 hours. There may also be a small drain to remove fluids from the site of the operation that will usually be removed the following day.

The catheter is important for the anastomoses to heal, so no matter how uncomfortable it might be, and how tempted you are to rip it out, leave it alone. Before discharge a nurse will instruct you on how to manage the catheter, and you will be given medications to ease the burden of having a catheter in.

Until you pass gas, you should not eat anything other than clear liquids. Once you do pass gas, you can start on a soft food diet (scrambled eggs, Jell-O, yogurt, oatmeal, toast). Your urologist will give you a variety of instructions. Please follow them because we want you to heal without complications. After a day or two, you should be able to resume eating a normal diet. You will be encouraged to get up and go for short walks. Walking limits the possibility of blood clots in your legs.

There may be complications. If you develop a fever above 101° or become nauseous, contact your physician. You may see pink tinged blood in your urine in the tube draining the catheter. This is normal. If you see dark red blood or blood clots, contact your urologist immediately. Major bleeding is not common either during or after surgery. However, sometimes a transfusion is necessary. Other reasons to contact your physician include shortness of breath or chest pain, there is no urine draining from the catheter, abdominal pain, or swelling in one leg or calf, or swelling or infection at the incisions (including any foul smelling incisions). Other complications that are nothing to be concerned about and not likely to arise, but which may seem alarming if they do, include:

- Bruising and or swelling of the scrotum lasting a week or two
- Swelling of your lower legs or ankles (as long as it is both legs or ankles, it is normal and can be alleviated by walking and elevating the legs)
- Bruising around the incisions
- Swollen abdomen
- Bladder spasms (a sudden need or constant urge to urinate)
- Discomfort in your perineal region (the space between your scrotum and anus (your doctor may provide you with a donut to sit on to reduce this discomfort).

It's important that you walk often and avoid heavy lifting or straining during bowel movements. Showers are okay but no bathing or swimming. Your urologist will instruct you on exercise and physical activity.

After the catheter is removed, a problem you may encounter is incontinence. After robotic prostatectomy some men are continent as soon as the catheter is out, while others will experience mild to moderate incontinence for 6-8 weeks. Your urologist will teach you Kegel exercises which strengthens the muscles around the urethra where the bladder is attached (anastomosis).

You can try Kegel's while you're peeing, and if the exercise stops the urinary flow, you're doing them correctly. Kegel's exercises are easy to learn. They're as simple as contracting your sphincter as if trying not to pass gas. During waking hours, try doing ten sets of ten, holding them for a count of ten. Some urologists recommend doing Kegel's in the weeks before your surgery in order to strengthen the sphincter muscle necessary for continence. Once the catheter is removed, try a few sets every day for the first few days, then steadily increase to ten sets every other hour for one week, then every hour until the incontinence is no longer a problem. (In the meantime, Depends for Men work well.)//

In rare cases, you may suffer bowel or blood vessel injury, blood clots in your legs and/or lungs, or a delayed return of your bowel function (ileus). Infections can be serious, but these complications are rare and occur in less than one percent of all prostatectomies.

Do not use tobacco or aspirin, do not tamper with your incisions or catheter, avoid strenuous activity but remain active (walking hourly and avoiding prolonged sitting), and contact your doctor right away if any problems arise.

In about two percent of radical prostatectomies, incontinence doesn't clear up after several months of time and Kegels. If incontinence is still a problem after a year, two surgical procedures can be done to fix it. One is an artificial sphincter and the other is a "urethra suspension" or "sling". These anti-incontinence procedures are successful most of the time.

Another major concern of most men is erectile dysfunction (ED) or impotence. I'm sorry guys, but it's true, 40 to 60 percent of men who undergo radical prostatectomies have some form of ED, ranging from mild to severe. The younger you are, the less likely you are to develop either ED or incontinence, and if you had healthy sexual functioning before surgery, you're less likely to develop an ED problem following prostate surgery. Most importantly, as I indicated earlier, the likelihood of developing ED is lessened if one or both of the neurovascular bundles (the nerves surrounding your prostate) are spared. The earlier a clinically significant cancer is discovered, and the smaller the cancer is, the better chance you have of have a server sparing prostatectomy. However, even the most experienced surgeon will not leave the nerves intact if the cancer is close to the nerves or even abuts the nerves. Your surgeon's main goal will be to eradicate the cancer.

Fortunately, there are many ways to treat ED, including effective drugs like sildenafil (Viagra). If you are unable to take ED drugs, or you don't respond to them, you might consider other methods including vacuum erection devices or penile implants (discussed in more detail in Chapter 12 on erectile dysfunction). As distressing as ED might be, I can assure you it's not nearly as bad as leaving your cancer untreated.

A prostatectomy is major surgery, and you will need time to recover. If your cancer is confined to the prostate, surgery is your best chance of being cured, forever. How do we know if it's confined to the prostate? The pre-operative MRI helps. If it looks like the cancer is confined to the prostate (T2) then you may be a good candidate for surgery. Once the prostate is out, the urologist will send your prostate and the seminal vesicles to a pathologist, who will examine the specimen. Infrequently, the pathologist will see that the grade and stage of the cancer is worse than what was present on the pre-op biopsy. That is because the pathologist will have the *entire* prostate and vesicles to examine, rather than just samples from the biopsies.

The pathologist looks for cancer at the margins of the specimen. Finding cancer cells at the margins increases the chances that the cancer may have spread outside the prostate. If cancer is found at the margins, it's called "margin positive" disease. This increases your chances of a recurrence locally (where the prostate used to be) or metastatic disease (meaning the cancer has metastasized to lymph nodes or bones). If the specimen shows margin positive disease, the urologist may refer you to a radiation specialist in cancer treatment (radiation oncologist) for radiation therapy. A PSA tests after surgery will indicate whether or not more treatment is needed.

Not all margin positive disease means the cancer will spread. Even if there is margin positive disease, cure is still possible. Margin positive disease means you're not out of the woods, and will need more active surveillance, if not additional treatment. Finally, if your surgeon finds that the cancer has spread to your lymph nodes, the survival rate isn't as good, but again, it does not necessarily mean a death sentence. It may mean that you will need additional therapy—such as radiation, hormone ablation or chemotherapy, to extend your life. https://pubmed.ncbi.nlm.nih.gov/9302141/

Six weeks after surgery, your PSA will be checked. If the cancer was limited to the prostate, the PSA will usually be undetectable

(<0.05). If PSA is noted, your doctor will discuss next steps. These steps will include checking PSAs every three to six months in the first year after surgery, and every six months to one year afterward. If PSA starts to rise above zero on subsequent tests, your cancer has recurred or had spread at the time of surgery. Your urologist, radiation oncologist and medical oncologist will consider options which may include radiation, hormone therapy, or chemotherapy. A lot of this decision making depends on new imaging techniques using special MRIs and PET/CT scans (PSMA scan) to find out where the cancer is.

Radiation Therapy

For many of the various stages and grades of prostate cancer, radiation is a good option. It may be that you are a good candidate for either radiation therapy or surgery. Or, because of the cancer stage, other medical problems, and other factors, radiation may be a better option than surgery. The bottom line is that radiation therapy works for prostate cancer.

Radiation may sound frightening, but for many men it may be the best option. The risks of radiation are different than surgery. Up until the latter half of the 20th century, radiation was considered harmless, yet many people suffered serious health complications related to being exposed to high levels of radiation. Our knowledge of the risks of radiation, however, combined with remarkable technological advances, have enabled us to now use reduced levels of radiation targeting tumors with precision while protecting the surrounding tissues. Thus, the damage radiation can cause—killing cells—can now be harnessed to kill only cancer cells.

Basically, there are two primary forms of radiation used to treat prostate cancer—External Beam Radiation Therapy (EBRT) and Brachytherapy. Brachytherapy involves planting radioactive "seeds" in your prostate. Let's begin with these seeds, a common treatment for some prostate cancers.

Brachytherapy is a procedure done on an outpatient basis. Although you will be given general anesthesia during the procedure, there is less recovery time and fewer risks when compared to a radical prostatectomy. To determine if you're a good candidate for brachytherapy or might be better suited to external beam therapy, you'll meet with a radiation oncologist—a physician who specializes in using radiation for cancer treatment. Men who have difficulty urinating, or urinary tract disorders, may not be good candidates. Also, if your cancer is one with high Gleason Score or advanced T2 or T3 stage, or your prostate is large (over 60 grams), brachytherapy may not be the best option. If you have minimal urinary tract symptoms, and if your cancer is considered low to intermediate risk, then you may be a good candidate for brachytherapy.

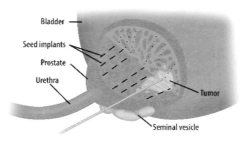

Brachytherapy for Prostate Cancer

There are two types of prostate brachytherapy, high dose and low dose. With high dose brachytherapy, high concentrations of radiation are directed into the prostate for just a few minutes. With low dose, radioactive seeds are left in the prostate to deliver low doses of radiation over many months, almost like a "time-release" radiation.

The preparation for either is similar to the preparation for a prostatectomy. You'll meet with your radiation oncologist, you'll have blood tests and a cardiac evaluation, and you'll have only liquids for 24-hours preceding the operation, and nothing the morning of surgery. Again, you'll have to stop taking aspirin or any blood thinners, and if you smoke, you should avoid tobacco products for a couple of weeks.

Pre-operative procedures may include a digital rectal exam and a cystoscopy (a small, flexible camera inserted through the urethra into the bladder), a proctosigmoidoscopy (a camera inserted through the rectum), and a transrectal ultrasound (through a probe inserted into the rectum). These procedures are necessary to determine the proper placement of the seeds. You'll also have a Foley catheter put into place to drain urine during and after the procedure.

For low-dose brachytherapy (LDR), needles containing radioactive seeds about the size of a grain of rice, are strategically inserted into the prostate through the perineum (the space between the scrotum and rectum). Because you'll be under anesthesia, you won't feel any pain and you will be discharged the same day. The seeds will remain in your prostate permanently, and though they are not high dose, you'll be asked to avoid children and pregnant women for a while afterwards, as well as use a condom during sex.

For high-dose brachytherapy (HDR), the radiation is delivered through wires that are passed through small tubes inserted into your prostate through the perineum under general anesthesia. After the tubes have been put into place and the general anesthesia wears off, you will be given a local anesthesia (often self-administered through a pump that you control). You'll have a post-operative CT scan to make any necessary adjustments in the placement of the tubes. This procedure will take about an hour, during which you'll be conscious, but anesthetized locally. After the CT scan, you will rest in bed two to three hours while the scans are analyzed, and your treatment plan is prepared. During this time, you will need to remain relatively still, changing positions only with the assistance of a nurse in order to ensure the tubes remain in place.

After the scans have been analyzed, high doses of radiation are delivered through the wires. Due to the high-level of radiation, you'll be alone in the treatment room during the procedure, which lasts about half an hour, but your treatment team will be continuously communicating with you throughout the procedure. The most discomforting aspect of the procedure is the need to remain still while the radiation is administered.

If you are only having one round of HDR, you should be able to go home at the end of the day, but if you need two or three rounds, you'll stay for two to three more days. There won't be any seeds left in your prostate with high-dose brachytherapy, and there will be no need to avoid children or pregnant women, as there will be no residual radiation in your body.

With either high-dose or low-dose, your perineal area maybe mildly to moderately sore for a few days, and you'll be advised to take over-the-counter pain medication and use ice packs to help the pain and swelling. The soreness will subside after a few days, and unlike a prostatectomy, you'll be able to resume your normal activities with minimal down time, though you may be advised to avoid heavy lifting and strenuous activities for a few days.

Your PSA will be checked when you return for your follow-up, but don't be alarmed if it is higher than pre-brachytherapy levels. It's not unusual for patients to experience a post-operative "bounce" in PSA following HDR, but the PSA usually declines sharply soon after. If PSA falls below 2 and stays there, the radiation treatment is considered effective.

The side effects and potential complications of LDR and HDR are different than with a prostatectomy. The most common complications include urinary problems, such as difficulty peeing, pain or discomfort with urination or in the perineal area, urgency and trouble emptying your bladder. Temporarily you may see blood in your urine, stool, or ejaculate. Bowel movements can be urgent and frequent. Unfortunately, some men undergoing brachytherapy will have erectile dysfunction. Fortunately, we now have effective treatments for ED discussed in chapter 12.

These side effects are all manageable and most (but not all) may resolve over time. Other potential risks of brachytherapy include bladder or rectum cancer brought on by the radiation, openings in the wall of the rectum caused by the radiation, or urethral narrowing. These risks are rare, however, and much less likely than the risk of your cancer metastasizing if you were to not have any therapy.

In some cases, radiation alone is insufficient. If your physicians consider your cancer to be high risk, they may recommend radiation combined with hormone ablation prior to radiation. For other high risk cancers brachytherapy is combined with external beam radiation.

External Beam Radiation Therapy (EBRT) is similar to getting X-rays, but more complex. Prior to EBRT three gold seeds are inserted adjacent the prostate using transracial ultrasound in a procedure that is similar to having a biopsy. These gold seeds serve as markers to target the radiation and allow maximizing the effect of the EBRT while minimizing damage to the surrounding tissue.

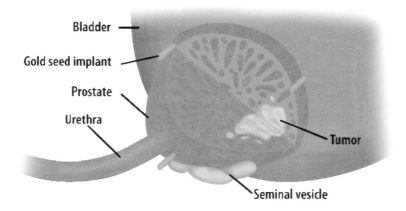

Transrectal Ultrasound Guided Gold Seed Placement prior to External Beam Radiation Therapy for Prostate Cancer

EBRT is done 5 days a week for 6-8 weeks. Because the prostate moves inside the body, a CT scan is done to exactly focus on the target (the prostate). You will lie down and be positioned, and the radiation machine will rotate around you while you remain still. You'll be conscious and not in any pain, and your team will communicate with you via camera and microphone during the procedure.

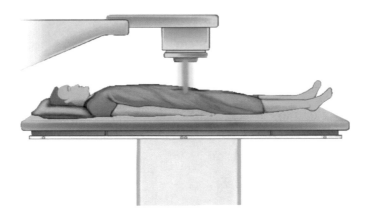

External Beam Radiation Therapy

It's becoming more common to do half as many treatments, about twenty treatments over a one-month period, but with higher doses of radiation, a treatment known as Moderate Hypofractionation. This treatment plan is often just as effective as the longer one. Another variation is Ultra Hypofractionation—five treatments of even higher doses of radiation. Both Moderate and Ultra Hypofractionation have fewer side effects than conventional EBRT, but with equal cure rates and less time commitment. Not everyone is a good candidate for hypofractionation, however. Your overall health, age, tumor stage and size, and other factors will determine if you are a good candidate.

If the radiation oncologist recommends a form of EBRT, the side effects are much the same as brachytherapy, but can also include skin disorders comparable to a sunburn, and fatigue. Secondary cancer from the radiation remains a risk.

In rare cases, your physician may recommend Tri-Modality Therapy, which is a combination of brachytherapy, external beam radiation, and hormone therapy. If you've had surgery, but your surgeon was unable to remove all the cancer cells, you may be advised to have some form of radiation therapy after surgery. Because there are many risks to doing surgery on radiated tissue, it is unlikely your physician will advise surgery *after* any form of radiation therapy, but very rarely this is also an option. The most common combination therapy is brachytherapy with external beam radiation, or some form of radiation therapy with hormone therapy (neoadjuvant hormone ablation).

Hormone Therapy

Since prostate cancer thrives on androgens—testosterone and dihydrotestosterone, lowering testosterone to castrate levels (<50), we can slow or stop the growth of the cancer. Castration is one way to eliminate 95% of testosterone, but pharmacologic lowering of testosterone, called "hormone ablation," is preferable for obvious reasons, plus it can be reversed, whereas once the testicles are removed there is no putting them back.

Hormone therapy alone is generally not a treatment option for localized prostate cancer. However, adding short term hormone therapy to radiation therapy improves cure rates for intermediate and high-risk prostate cancers. The aim is to irradiate and thus kill the cancer cells, while also weakening their ability to thrive through hormone therapy. The hormone treatment is usually a single shot every four months once or twice starting a few months before radiation.

Hormone ablation is the same as "chemical castration." Depriving your body of testosterone will slow or kill cancer cell growth. Plus, benign prostate glands will also stop growing. With little or no testosterone you will have a decreased sex drive, may experience hot flashes, weight gain, memory loss, erectile dysfunction, decline in muscle mass, increase in "bad" cholesterol, anemia, and osteoporosis (loss of bone density, which may lead to fractures). Hormone ablation is not something to be taken lightly, but it will delay or stop the progression of the cancer, sometimes for years. The side effects of hormone ablation can be made tolerable, and they may be temporary because once the hormone therapy is stopped, your testosterone may return to normal (this is called intermittent hormone deprivation therapy and I personally used it in 95% of my patients being treated for metastatic prostate cancer). Prolonged continuous hormone ablation can also lead to heart disease and diabetes.

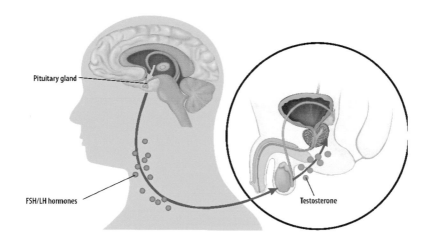

Androgen Ablation Therapy

Lupron and drugs like Lupron act on the pituitary gland by preventing the release of hormones (FSH and LH), that stimulate the testes to make testosterone. Testosterone stimulates the growth of benign and cancerous prostate cells.

Fortunately, if your physician does recommend that you compliment your radiation therapy with hormone therapy, or if you are on intermittent or continuous hormone ablation for metastatic prostate cancer, there are things you can do to minimize the side effects and risks: exercise;, eat a healthy diet low in red meat and high in fiber; and eat more plant-based foods (vegetables, legumes and fruits). Your physician can prescribe medications to mitigate the hot flashes (Depo-Provera worked well for my patients, SSRIs work (selective serotonin selective inhibitors SSRIs like Prozac/fluoxetine, as does Neurontin/gabapentin https://www.ncbi.nlm.nih.gov/pmc/articles/PMC3889979/), bone loss, and cholesterol. Acupuncture may be helpful in minimizing some of the symptoms, such as hot flashes. It's also important that your physician monitor your bone density if you undergo hormone ablation. To help with this problem, it's advised that you take 5,000 units of Vitamin D, and 1200 mg of calcium a day.

Ablative Therapy

One final treatment option for prostate cancer is Ablative Therapy, which destroys abnormal or cancerous tissues by freezing or heating the cells. There are two basic types of Ablative Therapies—**Cryotherapy** (freezing the cells) and **High Intensity Focused Ultrasound (HIFU)** (using ultrasound to delivery extreme heat to the cells).

If your physician feels you are *not* a good candidate for surgery or radiation therapy, or if you have tried radiation therapy and it has failed, s/he may recommend cryotherapy (also known as cryosurgery or cryoablation). Cryotherapy involves administering freezing gas to the cancer cells, which turns the prostate into a very cold ice cube, and thus kills the cancer cells. Cryotherapy is reasonable first line therapy for selected patients who are not good candidates for either radiation or surgery. It's also sometimes employed as "salvage therapy" in patients who have failed radiation.

Cryotherapy is done on an outpatient basis and begins much like brachytherapy, with you placed under general or spinal anesthesia. Needles are inserted into your prostate through the perineum. A warming catheter is inserted into your urethra to prevent your urethra getting too cold or injured during the procedure. Argon gas is then sent through the needles using a computer guide to ensure precise thermal delivery, while simultaneously monitoring the ice ball formation with ultrasound. Temperatures are monitored in several strategic locations around the prostate and urethra. As the prostate is cooled to very low temperatures, an ice ball is formed. Both benign and malignant cancer tissue is destroyed. As the ice ball "defrosts" during the procedure, the body's inflammatory response kicks in and the tissue is eventually replaced with scar.

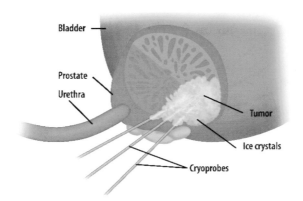

Cryoablation Therapy for Prostate Cancer

After the procedure you'll be discharged with a prescription for antibiotics and pain medication. Your physician may also prescribe tamsulosin (Flomax) to relax bladder internal sphincter so that once the catheter is removed in a week you'll find is easier to pee. You can shower and return to normal activities the next day (though you will be limited by the catheter).

When you return for a follow-up appointment in one week, your catheter will be removed and your urologist will check to see if you can pee without it. Ten percent of patients are unable to pee and must learn to insert a catheter every 4 to 6 hours, usually for a few days. I've performed over 150 cryoablations and can't remember one instance of urinary retention post-op that required intermittent catheterization. It all has to do with how patients are selected for the procedure, and how it's done. I also saw excellent cure rates with follow-up at 10 years.

One problem with cryoablation is that erectile dysfunction rates are high and can be permanent. Other temporary side effects include bladder spasms, blood in the urine, scrotal swelling, burning and irritation from the catheter, and numbness in the head of the penis. These side effects typically resolve with a few days or weeks.

In recent years technological advances have improved ablative therapy making it more precise, minimizing side effects. A technique called "Focal Therapy" targets just the tumor, and spares the part of the prostate that does not have cancer in it. Focal therapy, whether using radiation, cryotherapy, or HIFU, is still in it's infancy, and until imaging techniques are highly specific to allow accurate and complete targeting, these "Focal" procedures should be considered experimental. Before Focal Therapy becomes standard practice, however, results have to be as good or better than standard therapy, be it surgery, radiation, cryoablation, or HIFU, which we'll discuss next.

High Intensity Focused Ultrasound (HIFU) is one last treatment option you might consider if you have early-stage cancer or other methods have failed. HIFU has only recently been FDA approved, which means the treatment is still in its infancy, but the treatment does show some promise for certain patients.

After a probe is inserted into your rectum, high-intensity ultrasound waves are delivered to the affected tissues, thus delivering high blasts of heat to the cancer cells, killing them. The side effects are similar to those for cryotherapy. Because it's a relatively new treatment, the experience and skill of your surgeon can make a difference in the side effects that you might experience.

Fertility

Fertility is not an issue for most if not all men with prostate cancer, because 99% of men with prostate cancer are beyond the age of wanting children. However, if you've had a prostatectomy, and your seminal vesicles are removed you will no longer be fertile. The other therapies (radiation, cryotherapy, HIFU, and hormone ablation) also will likely render you infertile. Thus, if you do plan to have children following prostate therapy (which is rare) you should discuss methods of sperm preservation with your physician before treatment.

Genetic Markers for Early Detection of Prostate Cancer

It's at this point where exciting new data on genetic markers comes into play, particularly BRCA1 and BRCA2. You may have heard of BRCA1 and 2 if you know anyone who has had breast cancer. BRCA 1/2 are genes. Genes code for proteins. BRCA codes for a protein that suppresses tumor (cancer) growth. Mutations occur in these genes. The mutations can occur spontaneously, or they can be passed on from parent/grandparents to offspring. BRCA1 and 2 mutations are associated with an increased risk of breast and ovarian cancers. We are now finding that BRCA1 and 2 mutations are associated with other cancers, including prostate.

Another blood test that's increasing the accuracy of detecting high-grade disease is called circulating tumor cells or CTCs. CTCs are present in 60% of men with localized disease. When you combine genetic markers (BRCA and others), with mpMRI, and CTCs, there is over a 90% accuracy of detecting high grade disease[x]. Think about that for a minute. A 90% accuracy of detecting high grade disease is by far the best screening accuracy of *any* cancer that affects humans.

If you've just been diagnosed with prostate cancer, the decision you are about to make is difficult and complicated. One of the reasons I've written this chapter and this book is to help you work with your urologist to make the best decisions regarding your cancer. You need tools, data, facts, and an understanding of what prostate cancer involves and what treatment is available. It helps to know the benefits and risks of each type of therapy for which you are a candidate. Your urologist will help guide you through this maze, but ultimately it's your body and your life, and the decision is yours.

You and your cancer are unique, defined by your state of health, your age, your cancer stage and grade, and what's important to you. Your decision regarding what treatment to have, if any, depends on balancing risks—"If I do active surveillance, what's the risk that the cancer will grow, change, spread or metastasize? If I am not a candidate for Active Surveillance, what are my chances of being cured at 5,10, and 15 years if I choose surgery vs radiation? Depending on what therapy I have, what are my chances of having a recurrence? If I have a recurrence, can I be cured? How? What does that entail?"

I found that the better informed the patient, the better the decision. Confronted with the overwhelming amount of information, misinformation, and disinformation on the internet, it's hard for you to be informed well enough to make a good decision. Also, the conversation between you and your urologist takes time, a lot of time. Urologists are busy, and they may not have the time they'd like to spend with you. This chapter was written in hopes that this material will inform that discussion.

When considering the side effects of treatment, consider this, once the cancer has metastasized, there is no cure. There is palliative therapy like hormone ablation, radiation, and chemotherapy, but these therapies do not cure anyone with metastatic disease, and there are significant side effects associated with all of these palliative treatments.

Also consider this fact—prostate cancer is the second leading cause of cancer-related deaths among men, second only to lung cancer. Unlike lung cancer, you can't minimize your chances of getting it by avoiding any one thing, such as cigarettes. A healthy diet and exercise help, but I've seen many fit men who have a healthy diet and exercise die from prostate cancer or are miserable being on hormone ablation therapy. The most valuable step you can take is to keep an eye on your PSA and start checking it early (I recommend age 40 as I discuss in the previous chapter) If you've been diagnosed and treated for prostate cancer, or if you are on Active Surveillance, PSA is especially useful to assess how well you are doing. If you do recur, or if your cancer progresses, PSA tells us whether or not you need additional therapy.

Conclusion

The bottom line is that if your cancer is caught early (Stage T1 or T2), and treated early with either surgery or radiation, you have a 98% chance that after five years there will be no evidence of cancer, a 96% chance that after ten years you still won't have any evidence of cancer, and after 15 years a 94% chance that there will be no evidence of cancer (plus or minus 5%). What's more, if the cancer was detected and treated early, even if you aren't completely cured, your chances of surviving with your cancer are very high.

But if the cancer is not caught early and metastasizes to the bones or lymph nodes, or if there is a great amount of cancer outside the prostate, the average survival rate drops to 30% (after 5 years from the time of diagnosis). These statistics alone should convince you that PSA testing has changed the face of prostate cancer, as treatment can commence much earlier. Technological advances with the daVinci robot for radical prostatectomy and more specific and targeted radiation therapy, have improved treatment outcomes with fewer complications and better survival. With these new therapies combined with appropriate early detection, we are seeing fewer cases of metastatic disease, and fewer deaths.

I realize that this is a tough decision. Urologists want you to make the best decision that is in concert with your goals and values. If something doesn't seem right, don't hesitate to seek a second opinion. If your urologist is pushing surgery and hasn't discussed radiation, don't hesitate asking her/him for a referral to a radiation oncologist. It's okay to ask for a second opinion from another urologist. Most urologists welcome that request because they want you to make the right decision. I found that patients who were well informed and understood the risks and benefits of all the treatment options available to them, ultimately made a decision that we both thought was the best decision. After all, it's your life, and your body. Through shared-decision making, you're more likely to make the decision that is right for you.

CHAPTER 8

Your Scrotum and Testicles

The scrotum is both critical to the survival of our species, and alarmingly vulnerable. Every man has felt the excruciating pain of a whack to the scrotum, whether accidental or intended, just as he's felt the indescribable pleasure that same vulnerable part of our bodies brings us. For us urologists, the scrotum is less an engineering failure, than a fascinating feat of evolutionary engineering.

Scrotums contain the testes which make sperm and testosterone. Sperm leaves the testes and travels through a series of narrow, delicate tubes (the ductuli efferences), and enters the epididymis. The epididymis is not some Greek god but is instead over twenty feet of coiled thin tube that is the diameter of a couple of strands of hair. The epididymis is behind the testes and is about the size of a 2 inch caterpillar. Attached to this long bean shaped coil of tubing are two small appendages (no bigger than 1/16th of an inch) called the appendix testes and the appendix epididymis. In the embryo, these appendages are the precursors to the fallopian tubes in females. In males, their function is pretty much useless, unless one counts the business they bring us urologists when they become twisted and cause significant pain. But I'm getting ahead of myself. Let's get back to the voyage of the sperm.

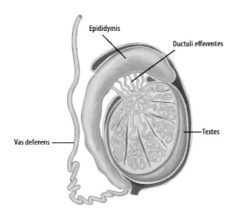

Scrotal Anatomy

At the bottom of the epididymis begins the vas deferens—Latin for "carrying away vessel" which carries the sperm to the prostate. Recall from Chapter 1 that these vas deferens are two tubes that leave the scrotum and pass along each side of the public bone into the groin. From there they circle down in the pelvis to join the seminal vesicles underneath the bladder to form the ejaculatory ducts. The ejaculatory ducts connect and drain into the prostate. Along the way, numerous problems may ensue.

Epididymitis

Every year in the United States, about 600,000 men, mostly between the ages of 15 and 40, are diagnosed with acute epididymitis—an infection of the epididymitis. The symptoms include pain in a sometimes swollen scrotum, which may be red and warm. The pain is usually limited to affected side. There can also be painful urination, urinary frequency, discharge from the penis and blood in the semen. Typically, the symptoms develop gradually, rather than suddenly. There may be fever. The pain can be severe, but over-the-counter pain medication (non-steroidal anti-inflammatory meds like Motrin or Advil) helps, as does keeping the scrotum cooled with an ice pack (frozen peas work great!).

If you develop symptoms of epididymitis, it's important to see a doctor. Some men ignore the symptoms, hoping the infection will clear up on its own. This is a mistake. Delayed treatment, or no treatment at all, can lead to an abscess or pocket of pus that may require surgical drainage, or even lead to needing to have the testes and epididymis removed. And though not common, delayed treatment can also cause infertility.

Once you do see a doctor, the first thing s/he will want to do is assess the cause of the pain and swelling of the epididymis. As with many infections, there can be many potential culprits. Although epididymitis is not, strictly speaking, a sexually transmitted disease, it can be caused by an STD, (namely gonorrhea, chlamydia, or urea plasma urealyticum). If you have bacterial epididymitis, you can transmit it to a sexual partner.

Acute epididymitis can also be caused by any bacteria that has access to the urinary tract, as well as mumps (which is a virus), or any obstruction within the epididymis, vas deferens, ejaculatory duct, or prostate.

If there is an obstruction or blockage between the epididymis and urethra, the back pressure from the obstruction can cause considerable inflammation, swelling and pain. The most common cause of obstruction is a vasectomy, though this complication occurs in just one to three percent of men undergoing vasectomy.

If you do not have an obvious urinary tract infection, or you haven't had recent surgery, or if there is no other reason to suspect a blockage (such as trauma typically from heavy lifting or a groin injury) your urologist may suspect a bacterial infection and prescribe antibiotics, even if a bug does not show up in a positive culture. In some cases, a couple of different antibiotics may be tried if the first fails to knock it out, because different bacteria respond to different antibiotics. The most common bacteria that cause epididymitis are sensitive to doxycycline, ciprofloxacin, and trimethoprim/sulfa. Whichever you are prescribed, take the full dose, which will be 10-14 days, even if your symptoms have cleared up—because the bacteria may still be there, and it's important to try and eradicate them.

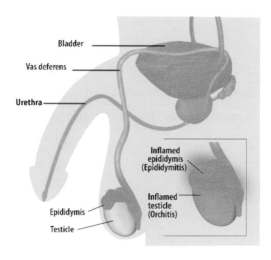

Bladder

Vas deferens

Urethra

Inflamed
epididymis
(Epididymitis)

Inflamed
testicle
(Orchitis)

Epididymis

Testicle

Epididymitis, chronic or acute

Once you begin taking the antibiotics, you should start feeling better in three to five days, though the pain can last for weeks and even months. Because bacteria may still be present, however, even once you're pain free, you should consult your doctor before resuming sexual activity, and ask whether or not your partner needs to be treated. If the epididymitis is caused by trauma or obstruction, it would not be something you'd transmit to your partner, and therefore your partner would not need to be treated.

One source of an infection in the scrotum is a virus that causes an infection in both the epididymis and testes. The virus is the mumps virus. In 1967 the vaccine for mumps was introduced and combined with the vaccine for measles and rubella, the MMR vaccine. This vaccine later became the MMRV vaccine in 1995 when the varicella (chicken pox) vaccine was added. As a result of these vaccines, cases of mumps became rare. When I was in grade school before the vaccine for mumps was invented, my friends who got it had puffy cheeks, fever, and missed a week of school. I was spared. It wasn't until I was in medical school that I learned that mumps can cause epididymitis.

Boys who have mumps have a one in three chance of having epididymitis. The resulting inflammation can lead to shrinking or atrophy of the testicle to such a degree that the testes shrinks to the size of a pea. Following a mumps infection with mumps epididymitis, the scrotum will appear "empty" because of the severe testicular scaring and atrophy (shrinkage). And, it's likely that the testes will no longer make testosterone or sperm. In addition, a common response seen in post-pubertal boys who have mumps is that antibodies form that attack not just the virus, but the testicular tissue itself. The combined outcome of all of this is infertility in later years. I've seen men who present with male infertility who had mumps during childhood or adolescence, and have tiny testicles due to mumps.

Sadly, despite the vaccines having virtually eliminated mumps from existence, with the rise in anti-vaccine sentiments and the misinformation around COVID vaccines, I'm afraid there may be a rise in mumps (like we are currently seeing with measles, and now even polio), and with it, more men will unnecessarily suffer the consequences of the decision to not vaccinate.

In some cases, acute epididymitis can become chronic epididymitis. The bacteria may have been eliminated but the pain and inflammation persist for three or more months. In these cases, non-steroidal anti-inflammatory medication may be prescribed for up to one month. And if that fails, on rare occasions, the epididymitis may have to be surgically removed. If chronic epididymitis is due to an obstruction, and the pain is not relieved by NSAIDs, either the obstruction needs to be relieved or reversed, or the epididymis removed.

Testicular Torsion

Testes torsion most commonly occurs in boy and young adults between the ages of 12 and 18, but it can occur at any age, even before birth. It is sometimes confused with epididymitis, however the pain associated with epididymitis will come on gradually, over the course of hours, whereas pain from testicular torsion is acute and comes on suddenly. Nausea and vomiting are sometimes seen with torsion, and rare with epididymitis. If you think you may have testicular torsion, time is of the essence, so if this is you, seek help in an urgent care center or E.R. immediately.

Testicular torsion means the cord that carries the blood vessels going to and from your testicle has twisted. The testes is suspended in the scrotum by the spermatic cord and the structures within it. If the attachments of the testes are faulty, it can turn and the cord becomes twisted, which cuts off the blood and oxygen to the testes and prevents blood from draining out of the testes. The testes can swell and the skin of the scrotum can become discolored. Torsion may cause the testes to change position and appear higher in the scrotum, and instead of hanging vertically, the testes will be oriented horizontally.

The pain can be so severe an examination may be out of the question. The key to diagnosing testicular torsion is scrotal ultrasound. A scrotal ultrasound uses sound waves to see inside the scrotum, and a doppler to measure the flow of blood. If torsion is confirmed (no blood flow to the testes seen on ultrasound), surgery is needed to un-twist the cord and attach the testes to the inner part of the scrotum so that it doesn't happen again.

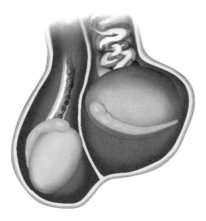

Testicular Torsion

A urologist will perform an orchidopexy (from the Latin term or-chid, which means gonad, and pexy, which means fix). This is done under general anesthesia. A horizontal incision is made through the scrotal skin layers to expose a blue or black testes and epididymis. S/he untwists the cord and the blood supply is restored. Once good blood supply is established, hopefully the testes will turn pink. If it turns pink, the teste isare viable (alive). The teste is then sutured to the lin-ing of the scrotal wall. The other testicle, being at risk, will also be fixed into place to prevent the same thing happening to that one. Unfortu-nately, if the torsion has been ongoing for 12 or more hours, the testes will not "pink up," and the likelihood of recovering sperm or testos-terone production is slim. The testes may even have to be removed in this case. The prolonged lack of oxygen to the affected testes may affect the fertility potential of the other testicle later in life, though that possibility remains subject to debate.

Chances are, should you or your son get testicular torsion loss of the testicle or infertility are uncommon, mainly because the pain from testicular torsion is so severe that few parents of boys wait to get help. The sooner blood supply and oxygen are restored to the testes, the better chance that testes will survive and produce normal sperm in testosterone down the road. So it's important to get help right away!//

Sometimes the scrotal ultrasound (or the physical exam) will show that the pain and swelling in the scrotum is coming from a twisted *appendix* testes or epididymis. If this is the case, you won't need surgery. Instead, you will be treated with a non-steroidal anti-inflammatory medication (Advil, Motrin), until the pain subsides. The twisted appendage usually disappears.

One final word about testicular torsion. Sometimes the testes can twist, and then spontaneously untwist. The acute pain will subside, and you might think you don't need to see a doctor. But you should, because the episode of acute pain might not be torsion, but something else. And, if it is a torsion that has untwisted on its own, it is likely to twist again in the future. So bottom line—if you or your son has acute scrotal pain and swelling, seek medical help right away. If it untwists and the pain and selling go away, still make an appointment to see what the problem is. If the urologist thinks that the cord has twisted and the untwisted spontaneously, he/she may suggest preventive surgery to keep the torsion from happening again.

Chronic Scrotal Pain

In the irreverent and sacrilegious musical, *The Book of Mormon*, the word scrotum is said more than 50 times, and 50 times, the word sends the audience into hysterics. When one of the African villagers declares that he's got "maggots" in his "scrotum," as the audience laughs, I cringe. I know that if you have a problem in your scrotum, you won't be laughing. In fact, until you figure out what is wrong, you're probably going to be pretty anxious. And if that problem persists, week after week, month after month, your chronic scrotal pain may occupy a lot of your daily thoughts.

If the pain has persisted for more than three months, you could have infectious chronic epididymitis. Your urologist will determine if this is the case with a good physical exam, a urine analysis and possibly an ultrasound.

If s/he rules out an infection, the problem might be caused by an obstruction. If you've had a vasectomy, you might be suffering from post-vas syndrome. One percent of men who have had vasectomies develop post-vas (or post-vasectomy) pain syndrome (PVPS), but you just might be in that unfortunate one percent. PVPS can be caused by obstruction and back pressure, infection, nerve compression or scar tissue, causing pain in your scrotum, pain or pressure with ejaculation, and/or pain during sex. If sperm leaks after the vasectomy, the inflammatory process that results can present as a painful lump called a sperm granuloma. Also, the back pressure following a vasectomy can result in micro-ruptures within the epididymis and chronic inflammatory epididymitis.

Fortunately, a post vas syndrome can usually be treated with over-the-counter pain medication (usually NAIDS). Sometimes physical therapy to strengthen the pelvic floor helps, and acupuncture has been effective. If those measures don't work and there is considerable inflammation or a painful sperm granuloma, it might be necessary to reverse the vasectomy or perform a surgical procedure to attach the vas to the epididymis (vasovasostomy or vasoepididymostomy). But suppose you haven't had a vasectomy and there's no sign of infection. Your primary care doctor has told you your exam is normal. If that's the case, you may have a varicocele—a bag of worms in your scrotum!

Benign Lumps and Bumps

If you feel a hard lump, mass, or bump in your scrotum, please don't hesitate to get it checked out. In many cases, it will turn out to be a benign lump, but if it's not benign, you want to get a diagnosis and started on a treatment plan. But first, let's consider some of the benign causes of scrotal lumps and bumps. One of the more common causes is a **varicocele,** or a bag of worms in the scrotum.

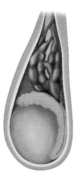

Varicocele

While it isn't a literal bag of worms, a varicocele is a tangle of varicose veins inside the scrotal sac (sometimes even affecting the scrotal wall). A varicocele is usually found on the left due to the anatomy of the internal spermatic vein that empties into the left renal vein and caused by a faulty valve between these two veins. If a varicocele is found in the right scrotum, or in both sides of the scrotum, the problem could be more serious and caused by something blocking the flow of blood in the right or both internal spermatic veins, so it's nothing to mess around with.

Varicoceles usually don't cause pain, and therefore some men don't even know they have them. It's only when a couple is having problems with infertility, and after an evaluation of the woman shows she isn't likely the cause of the problem that an exam of the man reveals the existence of this "bag of worms." A varicocele may be the cause of a decreased sperm count, abnormal sperm motility, and abnormal sperm. There are times when the exam is confusing and the urologist can't tell if a varicocele is present, but suspects one based on abnormal semen analysis, In this case a doppler ultrasound of the scrotum will confirm or rule out the diagnosis.

In most cases, however, a varicocele doesn't affect fertility, any more than it is likely to cause pain. But if you do have chronic scrotal pain, and you haven't had a vasectomy, a varicocele might be the cause.

A common "lump" in the scrotum is a **spermatocele,** which is a cyst that forms between the top of the testes and the head of the epididymis and can range in size from a few millimeters to larger than the testes itself. Three million men develop a spermatocele each year, most between the ages of 20 and 50. Like varicocele, spermatoceles may not cause pain, but sometimes they can. They are often detected on physical exam, or by self-exam. When the ductuli efferences, the small tubes that connect the testes to the epididymis, become dilated, a cyst will form. The cyst, or spermatocele, is filled with clear or cloudy fluid. It may contain sperm. Spermatoceles are benign. Your doctor will want to be sure that the mass is indeed a cyst and not solid, so s/he will want to shine a light through the cyst or obtain an ultrasound to be sure it's just a cyst. Occasionally a spermatocele will cause pain. If the pain isn't relieved with Advil/Motrin you may need surgery to remove it. The surgery itself is performed as an outpatient procedure under local or general anesthesia . When pain from a spermatocele is significant enough to warrant surgery, careful technique is required to preserve the blood supply to the testes and epididymis. Also, by removing a spermatocele, the passageway of sperm from the testes to epididymis may be interrupted and therefor affect the fertility from that testes.

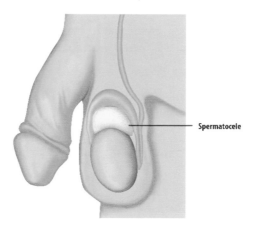

Spermatocele

Spermatocele

As discussed above, a lump in the scrotum caused by a leakage of sperm following a vasectomy is called a sperm granuloma. Sperm outside the transit tubes (vas or epididymis) is recognized by your body's immune system as something foreign. Your body's immune response is to form a **sperm granuloma** which feels like a pellet or pea where the sperm leakage has occurred. In some cases, a sperm granuloma will resolve without treatment, in others it simply stays there and doesn't cause problems. Occasionally a sperm granuloma can be painful and may need to be removed with a procedure like a vasectomy re-do, A sperm granuloma can sometimes serve as a bridge between the two ends of the cut vas after a vasectomy, in which case there will be sperm in the ejaculate following vasectomy. This is called "re-canalization" as there is a new canal between the two cut ends of the vas, and is one reason why vasectomies fail (1 out of 500 cases in the literature - more on this in the chapter on vasectomy).

Scrotal Swelling Without Pain

Sometimes your scrotum will swell noticeably without pain, or you may feel a "lump" inside. There are several explanations for scrotal swelling, as well as several causes for lumps and bumps inside the scrotum.

Hydrocele

A fluid filled sac that surround both the testes and epididymis is a hydrocele. The fluid is usually clear. In adults, a hydrocele can occur for no known reason, or it can be due to inflammation or injury. Hydrocoeles are usually painless unless they become very large, and usually do not require surgery. If a hydrocele is really big it may be unsightly or uncomfortable. I've had some patients complain that their scrotum touches the water when they sit on the toilet, a definite indication for surgery. Hydrocoele surgery is straightforward—the fluid is drained through an incision made in the scrotum and the excess hydroceles tissue is removed.

Five percent of infant boys are born with hydroceles. Most disappear during the first year of life. Hydroceles are made of the same tissue that lines the abdomen and are the result of the developing testes descending into the scrotum, taking along with it the lining of the abdominal cavity. By the age of one, the connection between the abdominal cavity and the scrotum closes off. If it doesn't, the one year old will have an indirect inguinal hernia/hydrocoele and is at risk for bowel getting stuck in the hernia, which can cause a significant problem if the blood supply to the bowel is compromised. If you have a one year old boy and he has a swollen scrotum the diagnosis may be hydrocele. In children, a hydrocele also means there is a hernia present and he will need surgery to fix it.

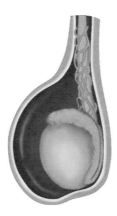

Hydrocele

Hernias (in men we call them "his-nias") can also cause scrotal swelling without pain. In adults a direct inguinal hernia is caused by a weakness in the abdominal wall. If this weakness develops near the public bone and the bowel or bladder migrate through the abdominal wall into the scrotum, the scrotum will appear swollen. These types of hernias do not resolve themselves on their own, and they worsen over time, so you will want to have an accurate diagnosis and arrange treatment. There are several modern surgical options using the DaVinci robot, laparoscopes, and mesh for scrotal hernias. These options are much better than how I learned how to fix these hernias 40 years ago.

Other conditions that might cause scrotal swelling include skin infections, lymphatic obstruction, or any medical condition that causes generalized body swelling (edema) such as congestive heart failure. If you notice scrotal swelling on one or both sides, be sure to see a physician to get it checked out.

Testicular Cancer

Testes cancer usually occurs in males from teenage years until they are 60, however more than half of testes cancers occur between the ages of 25 and 40. Undescended testes, even if they've been surgically brought down into the scrotum, is the most common risk factor. Family history also plays a role, as does HIV/AIDs.

It's a good idea for men of any age to know how to do a testicular self-exam. Doing so can detect small, otherwise unnoticeable lumps or bumps that could be a sign of testicular cancer. The best place to do a testicular self-exam is in a warm bath or shower, because the warm water allows the scrotum to relax. Using both hands, one to sta-bilize the testes and the other to feel the testes, roll the testicles be-tween your fingers. Remember, the testes are in front, and the epidi-dymis is in the back. You should be able to feel both. The consistency of the testes is kind of like a firm apricot. If there is a tumor or lump or cancer in the testicle, it will feel hard, like a rock. If you feel a lump or just experience a sense of "heaviness" in your scrotum, get it checked right away. Although there are solid benign tumors that oc-cur in the testes and epididymis, they are rare. Therefore, if you feel a hard lump or mass in your scrotum, please get it checked immedi-ately. The lump is considered cancer until proven otherwise.

Fortunately, testes cancer is one of the great success stories of modern medicine. The overall five-year survival rate for testes cancer in 95% (if you diagnose 100 men with testes cancer today, 95 will be alive in five years). Not all 95 will be totally cured, or cancer free, but they will be alive and living with testicular cancer. Those who are di-agnosed early, while the cancer is small and hasn't grown beyond the confines of the testes, do even better, and will experience a cure rate as high as 99%. Those men who present with a large tumor or one that has possibly spread, however, or those that have a very aggressive tu-mor, don't do as well. Early detection, diagnosis, and treatment are the keys to complete cure.

In addition to any lumps you might feel, symptoms of testicular cancer can include a sense of fullness in the abdomen or groin, pain in the testes or scrotum (although testes tumors are usually painless), back ache and even enlarged breasts (1% of testes tumors make hor-mones that cause breast enlargement, also known as gynecomastia).

If you have waited too long, you may have metastatic or late stage testes cancer. Symptoms of late stage testes cancer may include bone pain, low back pain, trouble breathing, chest pain, and cough (sometimes with blood).

If you are seeing a primary care provider for a testicular lump or mass, s/he will likely phone a urologist and get you in to be seen that day or the next day. If the PCP and urologist are suspicious of the diagnosis of testes cancer, they will send you for blood tests to include tumor markers specific for testes cancer. The PCP or urologist will usually order an emergency ultrasound of the scrotum to confirm the suspicion of a solid mass within the testes. Some urologists have an ultrasound machine in their office (they use it routinely for prostate biopsies) and may do the sonogram themselves.

Once the diagnosis of a probable malignancy in the testes is made, the urologist will schedule you for an urgent operation that requires removal of the testicle and spermatic cord up to where the cord enters the abdominal wall. This is done through an inguinal incision. The operation is called a *radical orchiectomy*. Hospitalization is usually not necessary, and you'll be able to go home the same day.

The pathologist will process the specimen and will tell us whether the lump is cancerous or benign, the exact size and appearance of the tumor to the naked eye, and what it looks like under the microscope. If it is a cancer, the pathologist will report what type of testes cancer it is, and whether or not it has spread outside of the testes into the epididymis or the spermatic cord with its' veins and lymphatics. Along with the tumor markers and other blood tests, this microscopic pathologic information is very important in determining the next steps.

Based on what the tumor looks like under the microscope, the pathologist will assign a type or name to the tumor—seminoma, embryonal cell carcinoma, teratoma (well differentiated or poorly differentiated), choriocarcinoma, or yolk sac. It can be confusing because there can be elements of each within each testes cancer. Sometimes a pathologist will say that the tumor is "pure seminoma" or "pure embryonal cell cancer." While these classifications may seem confusing to you, the pathologic classification and tumor markers are important in determining what happens next, and whether you will be treated with radiation, surgery, chemo, or a combination of all three. It goes without saying that the goal is to produce optimal survival and cure.

Testes cancer spreads from the testicle by direct extension to the epididymis and/or spermatic cord structures. Cancer cells can invade the lymph channels and veins of the spermatic cord. Lymph spread is specific to lymph nodes in the retroperitoneum that are situated along the aorta, vena cava, and iliac blood vessels in the pelvis. Spread of cancer via veins can show up in variety of organs, including lung, liver, brain, and bone.

Testes cancers are "staged" much like prostate, bladder, or kidney cancers, using TNM criteria (tumor, nodes, metastases). The stage of the tumor along with the microscopic cell type will determine whether chemotherapy, radiation, or more extensive surgery is indicated. To accurately stage your cancer, the urologist will obtain either a CT scan or MRI of the chest, abdomen, retroperitoneum, and pelvis after the radical orchiectomy. If there are neurologic symptoms, a CT or MRI of the head will be done also.

Once all this information is obtained, you will need to discuss options with your urologist, an oncologist, and radiation oncologist (radiation doctor and cancer expert). Frequently these specialists work together to formulate an optimal treatment plan. Sometimes there isn't one best optimal plan, and it's in this situation in which a shared decision making discussion can be helpful. *The goal is to produce the best cancer-free survival with the minimal amount of side effects from the radiation, surgery, and/or chemotherapy.*

Side effects shared by all of the treatments can include injury to organs in the abdomen, infertility, and erectile dysfunction. Each treatment is associated with other specific risks and potential side effects. The earlier testes cancer is diagnosed, the less chance there is of spread and the need for more surgery, radiation, or chemo. This is why a testicular self-exam an important routine for all men, just like breast self-exam for women. If you are diagnosed with testicular cancer, seek out a health care team skilled in treating men with testes cancer. There are many treatment options, and it can be complicated. I encourage you to engage in shared-decision making with an expert team. The sooner and more pro-actively you act, the less likely you'll suffer any long-term effects from testicular cancer, or the treatment of the cancer.

Conclusion

If there's one thing you've learned from this chapter, I hope it is that in most cases of scrotal swelling or pain, you won't have cancer. You may need immediate treatment, however, because you don't want to mess with inflammation or infection in your scrotum. And, if you suspect that you or your son might have testicular torsion, the sooner you are diagnosed and treated, the better chance you'll have of not losing your (or your son's) testes. The scrotum may be the source of giggles in comedy, but when it comes to the body, the scrotum is the source of fertility and the lifeblood of a heathy sex life. Take good care of your scrotum. And if you feel a lump or a bump, don't mess around.

CHAPTER 9

Bladder Cancer

If you are reading this chapter, you or someone you love probably has bladder cancer. In 2022 there will be over 80,000 new cases of bladder cancer in the U.S. That represents about 4.25% of new cases of cancers of all types. There will also be over 17,000 deaths from bladder cancer, which represents 2.8% of all cancer deaths. What's more, men with bladder cancer outnumber women three to one. Fortunately, bladder cancer has a high rate of survival. If you are diagnosed with bladder cancer (all types, grades, and stages) your five-year survival rate is 77% (2012-2018).

The bladder is a hollow organ that holds urine. There are three layers to the bladder wall—the lining or mucosa, which is a very thin layer of cells called "transitional cells," a layer of muscle (smooth muscle as opposed to skeletal muscle) and a covering outer layer called serosa. The lining layer of transitional cell mucosa extends from the bladder and lines both ureters, and the lining of the hollow portion of the kidneys where urine begins to collect before being transported down to the bladder via the ureters. Each ureter and the part of the urethra that goes through the prostate is also lined with transitional cells, as is the female urethra.

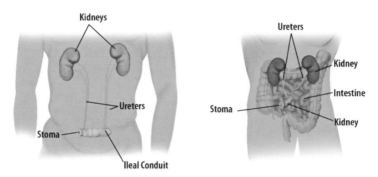

Urinary diversion, ileal loop (not continent, requires a bag or ileostomy to collect urine, which is worn on the abdomen)

When this transitional cell layer starts to grow out of control to form a tumor, it's called transitional cell cancer. There are benign tumors of the bladder, but these are less common, and the pathologist can tell the difference. Almost all (95%) cancers of the bladder are transitional cell cancers. Other bladder cancers are squamous cell cancers (3%) and adenocarcinomas (2%). Transitional cell cancers also occur in the ureters and the kidneys.

If you smoke cigarettes you are four times likely to develop bladder cancer. If you smoked previously, you are two times likely to get cancer compared to someone who has never smoked. The risk is the same for male and female smokers. Cigarette smoke carcinogens get into the bloodstream, and then excreted in urine. The urine containing the carcinogens sit in the bladder for hours in-between void, so it's no wonder smokers get bladder cancer. Other carcinogens like aromatic amines (hair dyes, diesel exhaust, and more) cause a variety of cancers including bladder cancer. Arsenic and aromatic hydrocarbons (coal, gasoline, coal tar pitch and asphalt) also play a role in causing bladder cancer.

I had several patients who worked as hairdressers with bladder cancer. A drug called cyclophosphamide which is used to treat lymphomas and leukemias among other things predisposes people to bladder cancer, as does a type of bladder infection with a bug called schistosomiasis, which is a parasite found in the Middle East, Africa, Asia, and parts of South America (this may present as squamous cell cancer of the bladder). Transitional cells cancers are more common in developed industrialized countries compared to developing countries where squamous cell and adenocarcinoma are more common. And external radiation to the pelvic area increases the risk of getting bladder cancer. In short, we are exposed to a number of carcinogens that may lead, over time, to bladder cancer.[xi]

Let's say you are the typical 60 year old male who without warning or symptoms peed blood. You call your primary care provider, and s/he schedules you for a CT urogram to be followed by an appointment with a urologist. The urologist will do a history and physical, looking for clues as to what may be causing the blood in your urine. You explain that you have no pain anywhere, and that you are urinating normally. But your urine is beet red and when s/he looks at it under the microscope there are sheets of red blood cells only, no sign of infection, no crystals that may indicate a stone. Maybe the CT scan shows a tumor in the bladder, maybe not. Your exam is normal (including a digital rectal exam showing a normal size prostate without firm or hard nodules). The urologist then says, "Let's take a look in your bladder and see where the blood may be coming from." So how is that done?

Cystoscopy is an outpatient procedure done with local anesthetic. It's not as bad as you might imagine. Xylocaine (Novocain) jelly is squirted into the urethra and held in place with a clamp behind the head of your penis. The longer the Xylocaine jelly stays in the urethra, the better it works (the urologist will leave it in for minimum 10 minutes and probably go do something else while you patiently wait). The flexible cystoscope is 5 mm in diameter (smaller than the normal male urethra which is 8 mm in diameter). There are three channels that make up the cystoscope: one for sterile water that flows through a channel; another for the fiber optic camera, which is part of the instrument; and a third to pass small 2mm wires or instruments. The fiberoptic lens/camera feeds into a monitor, so you can watch the whole procedure on TV.

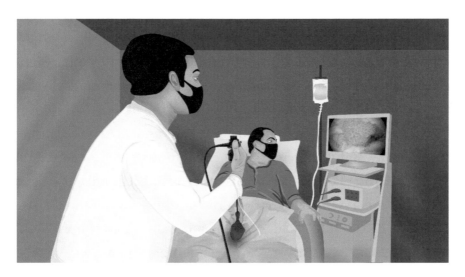

Male cystoscopy with a bladder tumor on monitor

The urologist will check to see that the urethra is normal, and then look closely within the

bladder for any abnormal growths. S/he will examine where the tubes draining the kidneys, the ureters, enter. These openings are called "ureteral orifices" and are situated on the floor of the bladder on a triangular shaped part of the bladder called the trigone. If a tumor is found, its location with respect to the ureteral orifices is important as you will see. If no abnormal growth is found, then s/he has effectively ruled out bladder cancer, provided there are no malignant cells noted by pathology. The visible blood in the urine is still without an explanation though, so the urologist will want to examine the urinary tract (ureters and internal collecting system of the kidneys) for a source for the bleeding. If, on the other hand, a bladder tumor is found, your doctor will tell you that you probably have bladder cancer. We have not yet come to the Shared Decision Making part yet, because under most circumstances the next step is to remove the tumor and look at it under the microscope.

The urologist will explain the procedure called a TURBT which stands for "transurethral resection of bladder tumor." Under general or spinal anesthesia, a scope is placed into the bladder. Using saline irrigation and bipolar energy (because it's safer than water and monopolar energy), the tumor is removed and the area from where the tumor is removed is cauterized. Several biopsies of the bladder lining are taken, and the biopsy sites are cauterized. The tissue is sent to a pathologist. Depending on the size of the tumor and whether or not there are multiple tumors, the procedure is usually 15-60 minutes. A catheter is placed and may be removed in the recovery room before you go home, or one or two days later, depending on the extent of the resection. This is step 1, but that doesn't mean you are out of the woods yet.

Once the pathology report is available, you'll go back to the urologist's office in a few days to discuss the next steps. Prior to that discussion, it's helpful to know something about cancer of the bladder.

Transitional Cell Cancer (TCCA) is graded much like other cancers, by the appearance of the cells and the way the cells are arranged. Grades 1, 2, and 3, correspond to the appearance under the microscope and correlate with how fast the cancer is growing and how likely the tumor is to grow outside the bladder and/or metastasize. Think of transitional cell cancers as either "high grade" (fast growing and likely to spread) or "low grade" (slow growing, unlikely to spread).

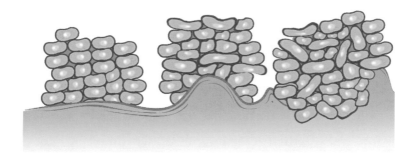

(L) Grade 1 Trasitional Cell Carcinoma
(M) Grade 2 Trasitional Cell Carcinoma
(R) Grade 3 Trasitional Cell Carcinoma

Like cancer of the prostate and kidney, the TNM staging system is used for bladder cancer. Recall T stands for tumor—the size and whether it's grown outside the bladder into the surrounding tissues; N stands for spread to lymph nodes; and M stands for metastasis.

To determine the T stage, your urologist will review the imaging studies and pathology report. Specifically, the pathologist will state whether the tumor has spread into the muscle layer or not. The TCCA will either be non-muscle invasive (NMIBC, non-muscle invasive bladder cancer) or muscle invasive (MIBC, muscle invasive bladder cancer).[xii] Let's assume you have a non-muscle invasive tumor, and following the TURBT you are urinating clear urine without problems. Your prognosis depends on the grade of the tumor, the size of the tumor, if there were multiple tumors, or if there are other abnormalities (variant histology) on the biopsies. Overall, for even for high grade NMIBC the prognosis is good with survival between 70% and 85% at 10 years. It's even better for low-grade well differentiated disease. The unfortunate thing is that 70% of TCCAs that are NMIBC will recur, and thus require more treatment. Depending on grade, 5-25% of NMIBC will progress to muscle invasive cancer despite multiple resections, chemotherapy, or immunotherapy instilled into the bladder. Rates of recurrence and progression correspond to whether the tumor is high or low grade, the presence of CIS (carcinoma in situ, a pathologic diagnosis of a flat tumor that is very aggressive), the T stage, and whether the tumors are multiple or solitary. In other words, bladder cancers are heterogeneous, and every situation needs to be uniquely addressed with the goals of preventing progression, loss of bladder, or loss of life.

After you've made it through step 1 (diagnosis) and step 2 (removal by resection, grading, and staging by pathology) you'll go on to step 3 for non-muscle invasive bladder cancer. Unlike Steps 1 and 2 which are the same for most everyone with NMIBC, step 3 can be extremely variable for each person. It depends on how the stage, grade, and other factors predict risk of progression and recurrence. Your risk of progression is either low, intermediate or high. If you are at low risk of recurrence and/or progression you will undergo cystoscopy every three months for the first year, every six months for the second year, and every year thereafter. If you have a recurrence, however, it's back to step 1.

For intermediate and high risk cancers the follow-up and surveillance are variable and more involved. If there is what's called "variant histology" present, the pathologist will note that in his report. Variant histology is the appearance of cells other than the standard transitional cancer cells. If you have variant histology, you immediately go into the high risk group, and there are multiple options that other high risk patients have, plus the option of partial or total removal of the bladder (discussed below). The risks and benefits of all treatment and surveillance options should be discussed with your urologist.

Immunotherapy and chemotherapy instilled into the bladder (intravesical therapy) work to prevent progression and recurrence in patients with intermediate and high risk disease. Immunotherapy is done with an agent called BCG. The chemotherapeutic agents are Mitomycin C and Gemcitabine. Sometimes these chemotherapeutic agents are introduced into the bladder immediately post operatively (after the original or subsequent resections) through a catheter.

BCG stands for Bacillus Calmette-Guérin. It is a live bacteria similar to the tuberculosis bug, but it doesn't cause an infection. When BCG is in contact with the bladder lining cells, it stimulates the body's immune system to seek out and kill cancer cells. Initial treatments are usually done in the urologist's office once a week for six weeks. During the treatment, your urologist will insert a catheter into your bladder, and inject the BCG through the catheter. Some protocols require maintenance therapy which is done every three months for a year and requires three weekly treatments during those three month intervals.

If there is no visible tumor on follow up cystoscopy, the urologist will want to make sure there is no cancer in the ureters or lining of the kidneys. After initial resection and staging, if blood in the urine persists, and there is no recurrence in the bladder, tumor markers in the urine and urine cytology (a "pap smear" of the urine) can be helpful in pointing toward the possibility of TCCA in the ureters or kidneys. Your urologist will have this in mind as s/he continues to monitor your cancer. Finally, there are newer methods available called "Blue Light Cystoscopy" and "Cxbladder" that have been shown to improve detection of bladder cancer that may not be seen on conventional white light cystoscopy.

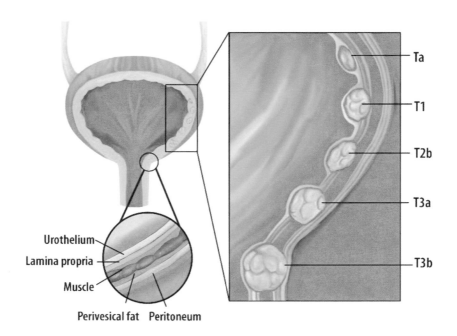

Stages of bladder cancer. Non-muscle invasive Ta and T1, muscle invasive T2 and T3.

After Step 1, if the pathology shows tumor has grown into the muscle layer of the bladder, the rules change. This is called muscle invasive bladder cancer, MIBC. Twenty-five percent of patients with bladder cancer will have muscle invasive disease. The risk of progression and metastases is high, so if your cancer has invaded the smooth muscle layer of the bladder, it's serious. If the cancer is invading muscle but confined to the bladder, the five year survival rate is 70% (that means 30% of people will not survive five years, even if the cancer is confined to the bladder and treated). If the cancer has spread to lymph nodes in the pelvis or adjacent organs, the five year survival rate drops to 38%, and if there are distant metastases, the survival rate is less than 10%. Sadly, these statistics have not significantly changed over several decades, but with a team approach to your treatment, you will enhance your chances of beating bladder cancer. You, along with your urologist, an oncologist, and a radiation therapist are part of the team. There are numerous treatment options, again depending on your particular grade and stage, and your life preferences definitely need to be taken into consideration. It's here that a Shared Decision Making Discussion is helpful.

Upon learning that you have MIBC, your urologist will want to further stage the cancer to see if has grown beyond the confines of the bladder, involves adjacent organs, tissue, lymph nodes, bones, or if you have distant spread to distant organs (such as lungs or liver). For this s/he will order a CT of your chest, abdomen, and pelvis (or an MRI), along with a bone scan. A variety of blood tests will be done to further assess your condition, with particular attention to your kidney and liver function.

Once the staging work-up is finished, you will know whether you have metastases or not. Then you will discuss your options. Let's assume that the muscle invasive bladder cancer is still confined to the bladder. In other words, based on imaging and blood tests there is no obvious spread to lymph nodes, no spread to bone, and no distant metastases. Guidelines for treating this disease have evolved during years of research and clinical studies with the goals of improving survival, while at the same time maintaining quality of life.

It used to be that the standard of care for non-metastatic muscle invasive bladder cancer was to proceed as soon as possible with Radical Cystectomy (removal of the bladder) along with removal of pelvic lymph nodes. The current recommendation, however, for patients in whom the cancer has not spread beyond the bladder or in lymph nodes, is adjuvant chemotherapy (chemo given *before* removal of the bladder). If the cancer is outside the bladder and/or in lymph nodes, a radical cystectomy may be done, and the chemotherapy is given after the surgery. Unlike prostate cancer, radiation therapy alone as curative treatment for bladder cancer is not an option.

And finally, if you do have distant metastases, the first course of therapy is chemotherapy. Your response to chemotherapy (the stage of the cancer after chemotherapy) and your overall state of health determines the next steps, which include surgery, radiation, more or different chemotherapy. This area of oncology is changing so rapidly due to the new "check point inhibitor" drugs that by the time you read this, whatever I write will be outdated, so we'll just leave it at that.

Radical Cystectomy and Urinary Diversion

A radical cystectomy in a man consists of complete removal of the bladder, the prostate, seminal vesicles, and the ends of the ureters (tubes that drain the kidneys). If you and your doctor decide that bladder removal or radical cystectomy is your best option, you'll want to be fully informed about what that entails. Chances are you'll wonder what's it really going to be like living without a bladder? First off, you'll be rid of the symptoms from the muscle invasive bladder cancer. No more peeing blood, or worse, passing blood clots, or even worse having those blood clots clog up the urethra, which has resulted in trips to the ER to get the clots irrigated out. If you've had bladder cancer, you've probably discovered that at times the bleeding has been so bad that you've had to be hospitalized after multiple trips to the ER and then OR to resect more tumor and stop the bleeding. Once your bladder is out, the bladder pain will be gone, as well as the horrible symptoms of having the constant urge to pee, being unable to hold it at times, the multiple trips to the bathroom every 30-60 minutes, getting up five to eight times at night to pee and getting no sleep. As bad as it might seem to live without a bladder, living with a bladder that has cancer in it can be an awful experience.

The operation can be done "open" through an incision that starts a few centimeters above the belly button and extends to the pubic bone, or through four to six small incisions using laparoscopes, usually with the aid of the daVinci robot. As more urologists are developing expertise using the robot, most laparoscopic radical cystectomies are being done robotically.

To prepare for the surgery, exercise and increase your caloric intake. If you're a smoker, you are at risk of pulmonary complications, as well as a variety of infections or bleeding. So this is a good time to quit. The day before surgery most surgeons will want you on a clear liquid diet. Some surgeons will also want you to do a bowel prep, but this varies from institution to institution, and even from surgeon to surgeon, so there is no one right way. If it's planned that you will have an urostomy (discussed below) or a catherizable stoma (also discussed below) it's often helpful to meet with a stomal therapist prior to surgery.

There are unique risks and benefits associated with a radical cystectomy. The main benefit to undergoing this major life changing operation is that it may be your best chance of being in the 70% of people with MIBC who are still alive in five years. The other benefit is, as I've already noted, that removing the bladder takes care of debilitating symptoms and bleeding from the cancer itself. Like most major surgeries there is the risk of bleeding, infection, damage to surrounding organs and blood vessels, blood clots, and heart and lung problems related to anesthesia and pre-existing conditions. It's a long operation lasting four to eight hours, and the longer the operation, the greater the risk. As in radical prostatectomy, impotence is a problem (and again depends on nerve sparing, which can be done for a radical cystectomy just as for a radical prostatectomy) and you will no longer be fertile. Then there are additional potential complications related to urinary tract reconstruction.

After the bladder has been removed, there has to be somewhere for the urine to go. In other words, the urinary tract minus the bladder, needs to be reconstructed. This reconstruction is also known as "urinary diversion."

There are two main types of urinary diversion, and several variations of these diversions. For our purposes we'll discuss urinary diversions as "continent" or "incontinent." An example of an incontinent urinary diversion is called an "ileal conduit" or "ileal loop." A type of continent diversion involves what's called a "neobladder" (new bladder). The neobladder can be attached (anastomosed) to your own urethra. Before attaching the ureters to the neobladder, the cut ends of the ureters are sent to the pathologist for a frozen section to make sure that there is no cancer in either ureter.

To create an ileal loop, a 12" segment of ilium (small intestine) is separated from the rest of the ilium. The two ends of the ilium are reconnected to reestablish the flow of small bowel contents. One end (the end furthest away from the large intestine) is closed (usually with staples) while the other end is left open. Each ureter (after a negative frozen section) is attached to the loop. The open end of the loop is attached to the skin and becomes the "stoma." A bag (ileostomy bag) is placed over the stoma. Once in place, urine drains from kidneys, down ureters, into the ileal loop, and into the bag.

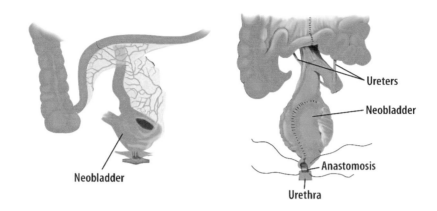

Ureters

Neobladder

Anastomosis

Urethra

Neobladder

Orthotopic Neobladder – "new bladder", usually constructed from a segment of small intestine (ileum). The neobladder is attached to the patient's own urethra and is called "orthotopic"

A continent (no bag needed to collect urine) type of urinary tract reconstruction involves the creation of a neobladder (new bladder). Ileum is again used, only this time a much longer segment is needed to create a pouch. The two ureters are connected to the pouch, and the neobladder is then attached to the urethra. Continence depends on the one remaining sphincter, the external sphincter. Because of body habits or internal anatomy, sometimes the neobladder cannot reach the external sphincter so attachment isn't possible. In this case, the pouch can be made "continent" by making a tube about the size of a straw that's formed from the same ileum and is part of the neobladder construction. This tube is attached to the skin in the lower abdomen, or umbilicus. With this type of continent neobladder, the pouch will need to be emptied by inserting a catheter every 2-6 hours to drain the urine.

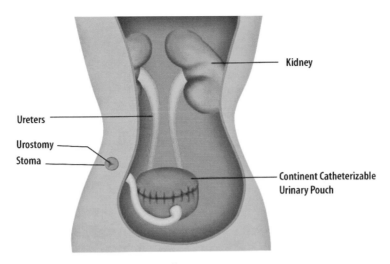

Kidney

Ureters

Urostomy Stoma

Continent Catheterizable Urinary Pouch

Continent urinary diversion (no bag, but must be catheterized several times a day to empty the pouch of urine)

The goals of urinary diversion are to preserve renal function and provide adequate urine drainage while at the same time minimizing complications. The benefits of a continent neobladder (either attached to skin, in which case it requires catheterization several times a day or attached to the urethra in which case you would pee in the normal way) are to minimize the impact on your body image, so you will not need to wear a bag to collect urine. The benefits of the ileal loop are that it's simple, quicker, and less likely to have problems. Your urologist will evaluate you to determine whether you're a good candidate for one or the other, based on your age and state of health.

Both types of diversion have potential complications in common. Whenever you make attachments, be it bowel to bowel, ureter to bowel, bowel to urethra, or even bowel to skin, those attachments can scar and become obstructed. The other thing that can happen is that the attachments can leak. Either problem may require another operation to fix.

Whenever you expose urine to bowel, there can be metabolic, acid-base, or electrolyte problems. Either type of diversion can be associated with renal deterioration. Both are associated with an increased risk of infection. In the case of a neobladder, if the pressure gets too high and the urine isn't emptied, the pouch can rupture. Last, sometimes the continence mechanism with each type of continent diversion will not keep a person perfectly dry.

There have been dramatic advances in creation of neobladders, continent diversions, and even the ileal loop, as urologists have learned how best to avoid these potential complications. I don't mean to deter you, just to inform you of the possibilities. Not all patients are candidates for neobladders or continent diversions. You will need to rely on the judgement and advice of your urologist.

Aside from having to catheterize and irrigate a cutaneous neobladder, your lifestyle should not be compromised. With an orthotopic neobladder (attached to your own urethra), your "internal new bladder" should be the same as if you have a normal bladder, except for the fact that you may need to periodically irrigate the mucous out to prevent blockage.

I normally don't recommend seeking anecdotal advice from the neighbor or relative who has gone through the same cancer ordeal that you are faced with. In the case of living without your bladder, however, it may be helpful for you to talk to other people who are living without their bladders. Your urologist will know of some of these people who s/he has operated on who are living normal active lives with either diversion. Ask them what it's like, what's involved, and if they would make the same decision if they had to do it again. I promise that this conversation will serve you well, and people who have gone through this are usually happy to help.

Conclusion

Bladder cancer is not necessarily a death sentence, there's a ray of hope down every avenue, no matter how serious the initial diagnosis is. It may take overcoming obstacles, surgery, chemo, and/or radiation, as all are possible treatments you'll may need. Like other chapters in this book, my aim in this chapter has been to help you discuss your options for therapy with your urologist, oncologist, and radiation oncologist through Shared Decision Making. Hopefully this chapter has provided you with information necessary to have such a conversation with your doctors.

CHAPTER 10

Everybody Must Get Stones

One of the most common questions I get asked on the golf course, at dinner parties, or anywhere where I'm introduced to a group of new people and they learn that I'm a urologist, will inevitably be about kidney stones. "I've had kidney stones about a dozen times," someone will say, "and let me tell you, they're worse than having a baby."

"Sorry to hear that," I'll say, as I try to focus on my golf shot or take a stab at my appetizer. "Are you still getting them?"

"Yeah, my urologist wants to blast them again. What do you think? Should I go ahead and have them blasted?"

"Hard to say," I'll reply as I make my shot or take a bite of my shrimp cocktail. "I'd have to see your medical records and X-rays, but . . ."

Everyone has a story about their kidney stones, or their husband's stones, their wife's stones, their in-law's, or friend's. Sometimes it seems like each one has a more involved stone story than the one that came before. It's conversations like these that leave me wondering why I didn't become a lawyer.

Fortunately, I love my profession, especially when it comes to treating patients with stones. It's really gratifying to relieve a person of horrible pain. Plus, we have all the good toys (lasers, shock wave lithotripsy, ultrasonic lithotripsy) at our disposal to treat stones.

I understand why so many people have questions. Having a kidney stone is usually an unforgettable experience. And they're common. About one in 11 people in the U.S. will have one or more stones in their lifetime, and up to one million people will visit an emergency room for kidney stones. And once you have—or suspect you have—one, you'll want to know what you can do to be rid of it. But all it takes is one Google search to realize there are millions of links to information about kidney stones. Even if a person has the time and ability to sort through this deluge of information, they're just as likely to find misinformation as useful information. While some of this information is harmless, some of it doesn't work, and some of it can be harmful. So in this chapter, I want to present you with enough information to make good choices with respect to diagnosis, treatment, and prevention. So just what are they?

An Overview of Kidney Stones

When we talk about "kidney stones" we're talking about a condition called urolithiasis—Greek for "urinary stones" (loosely translated). These "stones" are concentrations of crystals that can range from the size of a grain of sand up to the size of a tennis ball. I once removed a stone that size from the bladder of a 65 year old man. Stones smaller than 2mm usually don't get stuck, in fact, you may not even know you have one because you'll pass it without knowing. Urinary stones can develop almost anywhere in the urinary tract, including the kidneys, the prostate, and the bladder. What's more, they can occur in clusters—I once removed about 30 stones from a single kidney, and over 100 from a bladder!

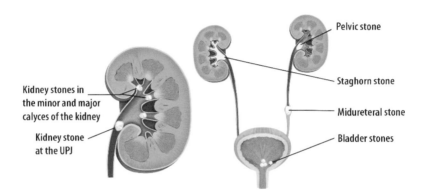

Possible location of urinary tract stones, also known as *urolithiasis*

While stones are common, who gets them varies greatly depending on climate, socioeconomic status and diet. There are also certain underlying conditions that predispose some people to developing stones. In developing countries, bladder stones are prevalent in children, largely due to dehydration and insufficient protein. In the United States, stones in children are less common (but they do occur), and more likely to occur in adults between the ages of 30 to 60. Men and women tend to get them in equal numbers, though the gender disparity varies. Stones afflict more people in the South and Southwest. The incidence is higher during warmer months due to dehydration, when urine is more concentrated. In fact, there is concern that climate change will lead to an increase in kidney stones as a rise in temperature leads to more dehydration. Thus, kidney stones are likely to remain a problem for many.

Symptoms

How do you know if you have a stone? If you've had one before, you probably know. If you haven't had one before, you may not even know it. If a stone is small (less than 2 or 3 mm), it may not cause symptoms (something we refer to as an asymptomatic stone). If it does cause symptoms, however, those symptoms can include intense pain, nausea, vomiting, fever and/or discolored or bloody urine. Let's take a look at these symptoms one at a time.

Kidney stone pain is usually in the flank, the area in your back just below the ribcage. The pain can be sharp and intense. It can be constant or come in waves. It can move around your side and into your groin and/or genital region. The pain is so distinct that we even have a name for it—renal colic—because it's a pain that will leave you crying.

The nature and character of the pain depends on the size of the stone, where it may be stuck, and if it is stuck, whether it is obstructing the urinary tract. The ureter drains urine from the kidney to the bladder. You have two ureters and each is about a foot long and the diameter of a pencil. So if the stone is tiny (say like a 2 mm grain of sand), it may not cause any pain at all. But a stone larger than 4 mm (a little over 1/8 of an inch) may hurt. As a stone gets closer to the bladder, it's more likely to pass spontaneously, but if it gets stuck in the part of the ureter closest to the kidney, it's less likely to pass spontaneously.

A stone lodged near the kidney that blocks the flow of urine down the ureter will cause increased pressure in the kidney. The pain from this increased pressure can affect your intestines, causing them to shut down. This is called an ileus, and it's effectively a paralysis of your intestines that causes the nausea and vomiting people with obstructing stones often have.

A stone that passes through the urinary tract can irritate the lining of the urinary tract. When this happens, you'll see discolored urine due to blood in the urine, which can appear light pink or dark as red wine. You may also see blood clots, or old blood, which will look like cola or coffee grounds. Sometimes the urine will appear normal to the naked eye, but a urinalysis will show microscopic blood, The urine under the microscope with be filled with red blood cells and sometimes the telltale crystals.

A most concerning symptom of stones is fever. An infected stone can cause fever—these are called struvite stones and are made of magnesium ammonium phosphate and bacteria. You can also have fever from a stone obstructing urine that is stagnant and infected. An obstructing stone and fever can be life threatening. If you have fever and flank pain (with or without discolored urine, nausea and vomiting) you should seek medical attention immediately. It may turn out that you simply have an infected kidney (pyelonephritis, discussed in Chapter 4), it could mean you have an infected stone, or an infection above the obstruction. A severe infection can lead to an abscess in the kidney. The greatest danger is when the infection gets into your bloodstream. This is called "sepsis" (in this case "urosepsis") and can result in shock ("septic shock"), and even death.

Whatever the symptoms, if you have a stone and don't pass it on your own quickly, you're going to need treatment. That treatment will depend on many variables, such as the size of the stone, the location of the stone, what the stone is made of (some stones like those made of uric acid can be dissolved, calcium stones cannot), the presence or absence of obstruction of the urinary tract (from the stone or other causes of obstruction), and whether the stone is single or are there multiple stones.

Treating Urinary Stones

If you listen to your parents or grandparents talk about stones, you're likely to hear about some archaic treatments. We've come a long way in the last four to five decades, and your options for treatment today are in some ways remarkable.

During the first part of my urology residency in the late seventies, we would do a variety of surgical procedures to remove stones from kidneys, ureters (the tubes that drain the kidneys into the bladder), bladders, and urethras. This was before lasers, shock waves, and ultrasonic lithotripters. Everything was done through an incision, what we called "open procedures." It wasn't until the later part of my residency in the early 80s that the subspecialty field of endourology—urological procedures done with minimally invasive techniques primarily through "scopes"—became accepted as a subspecialty within urology. Some older urologists who were comfortable with open procedures to remove stones coined the new practice as "end of urology." Some of them had trouble learning the new techniques, so for them it really was "the end of urology".

In 1985 I attended an AUA (American Urologic Association) meeting and sat in on a talk given by a German urologist who discussed a new technique to break up stones using shockwaves generated outside the body. The anesthetized patient was secured to a chair, which was then lowered into a tub of water. Shockwaves were generated from a device similar to a sparkplug into a thing that looked like a metal bowl. When the shockwaves hit the bowl they were reflected upward. The shape of the reflected shockwave was like an upside down ice cream cone. Using fluoroscopy (x-rays), the stone could be seen, and the special chair was moved to align the stone with the tip of the cone. No incision was involved. The shockwaves, focused on the stone, passed harmlessly through the body. The "sparkplug" generated a new shockwave with each heartbeat of the patient. The maximum force of the shockwave could be varied dependent on how hard the stone was. Thousands of these shockwaves could break up stones into tiny sand-sized particles that would pass harmlessly out of the body in the urine. We all sat there listening to this presentation totally astounded. Surgery using mirrors and hocus-pocus? Impossible. 40 years later, this technology, Extracorporeal (outside the body) Shock Wave Lithotripsy (breaking up the stone with shockwaves) is a mainstay treatment for millions of stone formers (though the large bathtub is not used very often anymore). Now there are special tables combined with fluoroscopy that can be moved from one outpatient surgical center to the next.

Technological advances continued into the mid and late 1980s. Procedures to treat patients with stones became less invasive, or even noninvasive. Endoscopes used to remove stones from the ureter and kidney went from being rigid to flexible. Optics and cameras improved. We learned how to employ double J stents to relieve any obstruction and aid in the passing of fragments.

By 1985 I went to special courses to learn some of these procedures that were not even in existence during my residency a few years earlier. I learned how to do a procedure we referred to as a **PERC**, which stands for percutaneous (through the skin) nephrostolithotomy (nephro—kidney; litho—stone; otomy—removal).

Recall from the anatomy chapter that the kidney is composed of a solid outer part that surrounds an inner or hollow part that collects urine. I used to explain it to my patients by telling them to think of the hollow part or the renal pelvis as a lake surrounded by a land mass (the renal parenchyma or the solid part of the kidney). The "lake" (renal pelvis) drains into a river (the ureter) that's about a foot long, which then drains into another lake (the bladder). Using fluoroscopy or ultrasound, a needle can be passed through a small 1 inch incision. The needle is then passed through the solid part of the kidney and into the collecting system and renal pelvis (the lake). Once the collecting system is accessed, a wire can be passed into the renal pelvis and down the ureter. The tissue from the skin to the collecting system (namely muscle and the solid part of the kidney) is dilated to create a "tract" about an inch in diameter. A hollow tube is then inserted into the kidney through the tract. If the stones are smaller than the tube, they are removed intact, and if larger, they are broken up using ultrasound, lasers, or other high-tech toys.

Imagine you are in the ER with kidney stone pain. The ER doctor has just taken a history, done a physical, sent your urine to the lab, and has obtained blood for several tests such as a complete blood count, an evaluation of your electrolytes (sodium, potassium, chloride), kidney function tests, and possibly a serum calcium, phosphorus, and uric acid assessment. As you wait patiently and in agony, s/he finally comes in and says, "I think you may have a kidney stone. I'd like to send you over for a CT scan." (If you are having fever and flank pain and are not in an ER or Urgent Care Clinic where they have rapid access to a CT scanner, but do have access to ultrasound, they might send you for an ultrasound first.)

Before the doctor sends you to get the CT scan, s/he will likely give you something for the pain, and possibly something for nausea. The CT scan will determine whether or not you have a stone and its location, but it probably won't be able to distinguish what type of stone it is, or its composition. That's important information in determining your treatment and how to prevent more stones from forming. (If you've had stones in the past, your physician may assume it's the same type of stone.) For now, let's assume this is your first stone.

If at this point your pain is controlled, you don't have fever, you are able to eat and drink, and your labs are all within normal limits (that is, no sign of infection, your electrolytes are normal, and your kidney function is normal). You may be sent home and an appointment with a urologist will be arranged within 24 hours. (If you have fever or an elevated white count or an obstructing stone, the urologist will be called in immediately and arrange to relieve the obstruction and/or remove the stone. If the ER docs can't control your pain, or if you are unable to eat or drink, the urologist will likely come in to take care of you and your stone.

But first, let's assume that you are feeling better and want to go home. You've been in the ER since 3 pm, and it's now 3 am. You've been told that you have a stone stuck in the tube between your kidney and bladder, and you have an appointment to see a urologist the next day. What happens next depends on four things—the size of the stone(s), the location, how much blockage is present, and how you are feeling. After a discussion of those variables, you and your urologist will jointly make a decision about what to do based on the probability of how likely you are to pass the stone on your own. This situation is unique to every patient with kidney stone(s). There may not be a single right answer, but a urologist with experience in taking care of kidney stone patients usually has a pretty good idea about which ones will pass on their own, and which ones s/he will have to treat. The first decision is, "should we intervene, or wait and see if it will pass on its own?" Again, this a highly variable, and there is no absolute right way of doing things.

Let's also assume your urologist tells you that you have a greater than 90% chance of passing the stone spontaneously within the next two weeks and gives you a prescription for medicine that will relax the ureteral spasm, which may help the stone pass spontaneously. S/he also sends you home with a urine strainer and instructs you to pee through the strainer until you pass the stone, and tells you to drink lots of water. Your urologist may also assure you that once the stone is in the bladder, it won't hurt when you ultimately pee it out. A 4-5 mm stone is about the size of a match head, and s/he will tell you to look for it in the strainer.

You go home with your strainer and meds and get on the internet to see if there is anything more you can do to help pass the stone. *Beware of misinformation.* We want you to stay hydrated, but there is no evidence that drinking huge amounts of fluids (more than a gallon or

3.5 liters) helps expel the stone. In fact, drinking huge amounts of water can actually be harmful because it can lower your sodium and potassium levels in your blood. (Later, we'll discuss the importance of water drinking in terms of prevention of new stones from forming.)

While browsing the internet, you're likely to come across claims like, "lemon juice (vitamin C or citric acid) will break down kidney stones." Lemon juice will not dissolve most common (calcium oxalate) stones. However, lemon juice (lots of it) or citrate may help prevent certain types of stones from forming. "Olive oil helps with the flushing process" another site will claim. Again, there's no evidence for that. "Most stones will pass on their own within a few hours to a few days." Again, more misleading information. You know by now that passing a stone depends on the size and the location. Some people are misled by claims that "cranberry juice is good for your urinary tract, so it must be good if you have a kidney stone." While cranberry juice has been shown to be helpful for urinary tract infections, as we'll see soon, it could actually add to the creation of new stones, and it's something we tell recurrent stone formers to *avoid*.

The bottom line is, take your medication, and if all goes well, the stone (depending on size and location) will pass. Be sure to use your strainer. The stone that shows up in the strainer might look like a BB, it may be rough or smooth. It can be black, brown, or yellow. Why save the stone? It's not because it's a keepsake. The reason we want you to save the stone is so we can tell what type it is, which can help determine how to prevent future stones from forming. If more stones do form, your urologist will have a better idea of how to treat you. I'll return to this point at the end of the chapter, but for now, let's consider what happens if you don't pass the stone. //

225

Let's imagine that you've gone home, waited for two weeks, yet still haven't passed the stone. You're tired of peeing through a strainer and you've had intermittent flank pain that's making it impossible to work or think of anything else. You've been back to the ER once, where they repeated the CT scan. You've been taking opioids to control the pain and haven't eaten much. You are sick of it and just want the ordeal to be over. "Get this damn thing out of me!" you beg.

In this situation, the stone is probably stuck. Although blockage can occur anywhere along the course of the ureter, there are three places where larger stones typically get stuck and obstruct: the junction of the kidney (renal pelvis) and ureter (ureteropelvic junction); 2/3 of the way down the ureter where the ureter crosses the iliac vessels in the pelvis; and the junction of the ureter and bladder (ureterovesical junction)

A general rule is that the larger the stone and/or the closer to the kidney it is, the more likely an intervention is required to relieve the blockage and pain. Stones larger than 6 or 7 mm are much less likely to pass on their own and often become lodged in your urinary tract. If the stone is moderate size (4-7 mm, which is about 1/15 of an inch to a quarter inch), and causing blockage and pain, you might consider a **stent**. Stents are soft plastic tubes about 2 mm in diameter. The center or lumen of the tube is hollow like a straw. There are tiny holes up and down the course of the tube. There are two J shaped curls on each end of the stent. One end curls up in the collecting system of the kidney and the other end curls in the bladder so the stent can't migrate either out of the kidney and down the ureter or conversely out of the bladder and up toward the kidney. Some urologists will place these stents under general anesthesia. Others will place them under local with conscious sedation. Stones of moderate size may pass spontaneously after two weeks of an indwelling stent, which is easily removed under local anesthesia in the office via flexible cystoscopy.

If the stone is larger than 6 mm, a procedure to break the stone up, or remove the stone is likely necessary. Placing a JJ stent before any stone procedure has the advantage of relieving the obstruction and the pain. An added benefit is that the stent passively dilates the ureter, which makes future procedures safer with better outcomes than not having a stent. These benefits are in exchange for possible minor discomfort from the stent. Some patients tolerate stents very well and don't even know that the stent is there, while others can experience bladder discomfort, frequent or painful urination, or possible pain in the kidney with urination. Pain in the kidney with urination while a stent is in place happens because during urination the pressure in the bladder is felt in the kidney since the two are connected by the stent. When you pee the pressure increases, which can cause discomfort in the kidney. This is not common, and the pain from a stent is usually nowhere near the amount of pain from the stone. However, with a stent there is also the risk of a urinary tract infection.

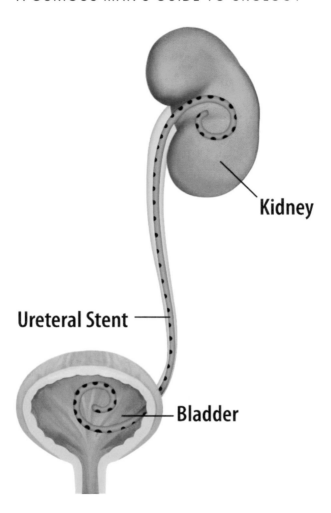

Double J stent

If your urologist feels that spontaneous passage is unlikely, then there are a variety of techniques designed either to break the stone up into small fragments, sand-like particles, or dust. The instruments that are designed to break a stone up are passed through a scope. The scope that is designed to break a stone up in the ureter is called a ureteroscope, and the procedure is called uretroscopic lithotripsy. The ureteroscope is a thin (about 4-5 mm) flexible fiberoptic scope passed through the urethra, then bladder, and then into the ureter. The image from the camera part of the ureteroscope is viewed on a TV monitor. Under vision a variety of thin, flexible laser fibers are passed through the scope. The urologist controls and sets the frequency of the laser impulses and energy that goes through the fiber that results in breaking of the stone into small particles or dust. Following the procedure, a JJ stent may be necessary for a week or two to allow the swelling in the ureter to go down and also for any small fragments to pass.

Another technique for breaking up a stone in the ureter is the procedure I learned to do in the mid-eighties—**Shock Wave Lithotripsy.** As discussed above, the shockwave is like an upside down ice cream cone. (Since shock waves pass harmlessly through water and since your body is 90% water, they are harmless.) The shockwaves correspond exactly (within 1 or 2 mm) to the location of the stone. Every time your heart beats another shockwave is triggered. The urologist can vary strength or intensity of the shockwave depending on where the stone is, the size, and whether or not it appears particularly hard. Shockwaves break the stone into small fragments. The larger the stone, the bigger the fragments and the larger the stone, the more shocks are needed. Usually, a double J stent is placed prior to the procedure, which both aids the urologist in locating the stone with fluoroscopy (x-rays) and helps the fragments pass once the stent is removed (though small fragments can also pass with the stent in place).

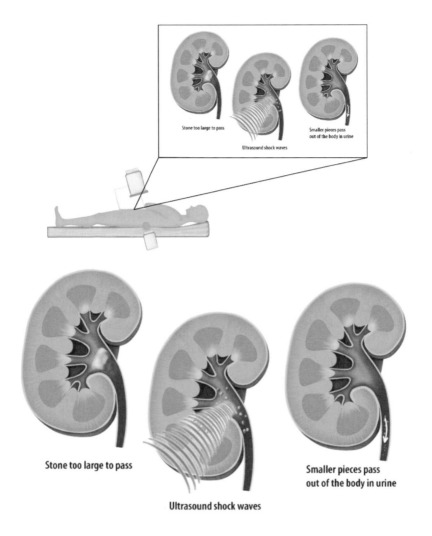

Stone too large to pass

Ultrasound shock waves

Smaller pieces pass
out of the body in urine

Extracorporeal Shock Wave Lithotripsy – ESWL

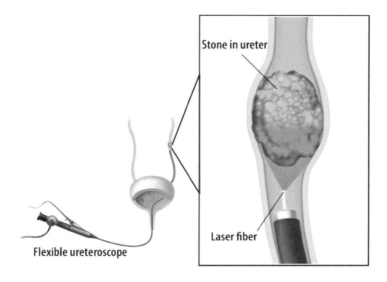

Ureteroscopic ureterolithotomy using flexible ureteroscope and a variety of different lasers that turn the stone into tiny fragments, sand, or dust.

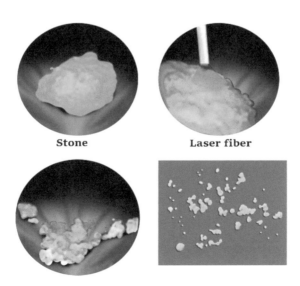

Stone fragments after laser lithotripsy

Either of these procedures— ureteroscopic lithotripsy or **Extra-corporeal Shock Wave Lithotripsy** (**ESWL**)—can be done for both stones in the ureter or the actual kidney. The decision to do one or the other procedure is a matter of weighing risks and benefits. The two procedures share similar risks and benefits, but there are also a different set of risks and potential complications associated with each. Depending on the size, location, and how hard the stone is, ureteroscopic lithotripsy (usually with a laser) may have an advantage over ESWL in getting you "stone free" (which is another way of saying "cured of your stone"), however, since ureteroscopic lithotripsy is more invasive than ESWL, the risk of injuring the ureter or kidney for example, may be greater. On the other hand, ESWL has a greater chance of leaving residual fragments. This discussion may vary from one urologist to the next based on experience, personal bias, and what tools the urologist has available. You may choose to have the less invasive (ESWL) procedure in exchange for the possibility of needing a second ESWL for residual fragments, or you may opt for ureteroscopy, because even though the risks may be higher, there's a better chance of you being stone free after one procedure. A good shared decision making discussion with your urologist often helps with this decision. Last, if the stone is small enough, or if the ureter has been dilated, the stone can be removed intact using a "stone basket" passed through the ureteroscope.

There are two instances in which a different intervention is necessary. Sometimes the stone is so stuck, and the swelling is so severe that the urologist can't relieve the obstruction. Another situation is when there is a significant obstruction with a severe infection, sometimes with a high fever, sometimes even septic shock. In this case, a radiologist can pass a nephrostomy tube into the kidney using ultrasound and/or x-rays. The tube drains the kidney and the infected, obstructed urine, and allows the doctors to relieve pressure in the kidney. Once the patient is stable, the infection treated, the shock and sepsis resolved, the urologist can then address the stone(s) that caused all the problems.

Stones in the Kidneys

Thus far we've mainly been discussing stones in the ureter. Stones can form in the kidney and remain there without causing any symptoms, even if quite large. On the other hand, if the stones in the kidney block the flow of urine, it's going to hurt. Stones in the kidney can also cause bleeding and infection.

Stones in the kidney can be treated in a similar fashion to stones in the ureter—with ureteroscopy or ESWL. If the stones are large (greater than 1.0 cm for some urologists), multiple, in the lower portion of the kidney, or "trapped" in a portion of the kidney, then the fragments created after ESWL have a low probability of passing. In this case, ESWL is not a good idea. Similarly, if the stone is in a tough place to get to with a ureteroscope, you may want to consider a different procedure. The same holds true for very large (> 2 cm) and multiple stones. It's not that ureteroscopy in these circumstances can't be done, it's just that the procedure could take hours and you still may not be stone free at the end. An alternative minimally invasive procedure in these cases is a percutaneous (through the skin) nephrosto (through the kidney) lithotomy (remove the stone) or PNL.

Prior to finishing my residency in 1982, procedures for extremely large and stag horn calculi (a large, branched kidney stone, sometimes infected) were done via a foot-long open incision. Once the kidney was exposed, we had to bivalve it like opening a clam (anatrophic nephrolithotomy) or open the renal pelvis (pyelolithotomy) in order to extract the large stone(s). For multiple stones in the kidney, we did a different open procedure called a "coagulum pyelolithotomy" in which we injected a solution that would form a cast-like jelly clot around the stones, which we then removed. Percutaneous Nephrostolithotomy (PNL) has rendered those invasive open procedures virtually obsolete.

If you and your urologist decide a PNL is best, you are put under general anesthesia. A catheter is placed in the ureter. Radiographic dye (to which is added a blue dye called methylene blue) is infused through the catheter in the ureter. You are positioned face down or on your side on the operating table. A one-inch incision is made in the back and a needle is inserted into the kidney under fluoroscopic or ultrasound guidance. Once the needle enters the kidney, a blue dye is infused into the kidney. A wire is advanced through the needle and guided down the ureter. A special balloon-dilating catheter is passed over the wire into the kidney, the tract is dilated to about an inch in diameter and a hollow tube is passed over the balloon dilating catheter and into the kidney. Through that tube, a rigid or flexible endoscope is passed and the stone is removed whole (if it's less than 1.0 cm) or broken into smaller fragments using either ultrasound (like a hollow jack hammer with suction) or lasers. Once all of the stones are removed, a nephrostomy tube is put into place in case there is post-op bleeding, residual stones in the kidney, or obstructing stones in the ureter. The following day, a CT scan is done to be sure all of the stone and fragments have been removed. If not, the nephrostomy tube enables us to look back in the kidney a few days later and remove whatever is left. If the kidney is "clean," the nephrostomy tube is clamped and then removed the next day and you are discharged home.

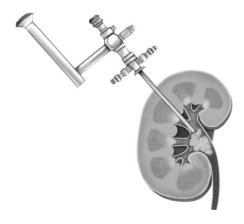

PNL

Percutaneous Nephrostolithotomy done through a 1" incision in the back through a rigid nephroscope for a large stone in the renal pelvis. A variety of different energy sources (ultrasound, lasers, etc) are used to break the stone (s) up.

In my opinion, PNLs are technically demanding. The procedure can be difficult for many reasons, and complications include bleeding, incomplete removal of the stones, infection, injury to the kidney, and even a collapsed lung (pneumothorax). So you want to be sure that if your urologist is recommending this procedure that s/he has discussed the alternatives and potential complications of all the procedures that are possible. And you want to be sure that the person who is doing the PNL has significant training, experience, and success with the procedure. Don't be afraid to ask. An experienced and skilled urologist will have no trouble answering any questions you may have.

Prevention

If you've ever recovered from a kidney stone, you've likely made it through level one of Dante's journey through stone hell. Congratulations. Hopefully as you read this you are stone free—that is, there are no stones anywhere in your urinary tract. The stones have all been removed or you've passed them. What comes next is important because for the most common calcium containing stones, you have a 50% chance of getting another stone within the next five years. Most people do *not* want to have to go through this again. The risk of recurrent stones is even higher if you have other medical conditions like gout, hyperparathyroidism, obesity, or diabetes.

After you've passed the stone or have had the stone successfully treated, your urologist will send the stone or fragments to the lab for analysis to learn what type stone it is. Several lab tests will also have already been done or will be done to rule out some of the medical conditions that predispose people to forming stones. Knowing these two bits of information—the type of stone, and any underlying medical condition predisposing you to developing stones—will aid your urologist in helping you to prevent getting more stones.

When talking about prevention, stone type is a good place to start. Since calcium oxalate is the most common type stone affecting 75% of first time stone formers, we will start our discussion with that.

Stones are basically crystals. About three-quarters of stones are made of calcium, either calcium oxalate or calcium phosphate. A more rare calcium stone is calcium carbonate. The common calcium oxalate stone can be made up of monohydrate or dihydrate crystals. Monohydrate stones are typically harder than others, which means they are harder to break up with the variety of energy sources your urologist will use (lasers, ultrasound, or shockwaves). **These calcium stones cannot be dissolved with diet or medication.**

About 15% of stones are **uric acid stones**. Uric acid stones are generally softer than calcium stones and do not show up on regular x-rays. They are seen on ultrasound, CT scans and MRI. Because uric acid is a byproduct of an organic compound called purine, if you have uric acid stones you'll want to avoid foods high in purine—beef, poultry, eggs, fish and organ meats. Thus, unlike calcium oxalate stones, there are dietary measures and medications you can take to help dissolve the stones. People with gout can form uric acid stones, and there are medications available to lower uric acid in the blood, which helps both gout and prevents new uric acid stones.

Another even less common stone is called a **struvite stone.** Struvite stones comprise about ten percent of all stones, and are made of magnesium, ammonium, and phosphate. Struvite stones are associated with urinary tract infections. The bacteria causing the infection produce an enzyme called urease, which splits urea to produce ammonia. As the urine becomes less acidic or more alkaline, the urinary tract becomes a favorable environment for the formation of struvite crystals.

There is an inherited disorder that makes prevention crucial. Cystinuria is a rare form of inherited stone disease seen in 1 of 10,000 people. Cysteine and cystine are amino acids containing sulfur. Like all amino acids found in blood, they are filtered by the kidney and then reabsorbed by the kidney and returned to the bloodstream. People with this inherited disorder can't reabsorb cysteine or cystine and since the two molecules are not soluble, crystals and stones form. The less hydrated a person is, the greater a stone will form (which is true of all stones).

If one of your parents had one cystinuria gene, then your chances of inheriting this one gene is 50%. If both parents have one cystinuria gene, then your chance of having both genes (homozygote) is 25%, and one gene 50% (heterozygote). The genetic defect is that people who have it excrete a lot of cysteine in their urine (100mg/day for one gene heterozygotes, and 1,000 mg/day for homozygotes).

People diagnosed with cystine stones typically are recurrent stone formers. If you are one of these people, you would most likely benefit from a consultation with a dietician to be sure you are doing everything you can to prevent more stones. It will also benefit your family and offspring to seek genetic counseling.

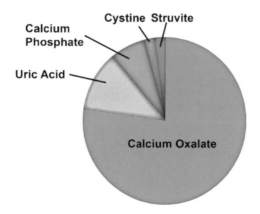

Not all stones are calcium oxalate. Note that uric acid and cystine stones are not seen on routine x-rays, but are seen on CT.

Now that you get a picture of the different stone types it's time to do something to keep them from coming back. The most common stone, calcium oxalate, forms because the urine is too concentrated, which allows the crystals to grow. While drinking lots of water won't necessarily help you to pass a stone, staying hydrated will help prevent new stones from forming. Staying hydrated throughout the day is the most important thing you can do, and you can start doing it now. You want to drink enough water so that your urine is clear to light colored, which means at least eight glasses a day. I recommend the "water drinking rule of 2" to my patients—2 8 ounce glasses first thing in the morning, a glass with each meal, a glass 2 hours after each meal, and 2 glasses at bedtime. That's 10 glasses a day. Most people who drink this much water will have to get up at least once a night to pee. Have another glass then. Adding lemon or lime to your water may also help, because the citrate in the lemon or lime juice prevents calcium oxalate precipitation in the urine. Lemonade can significantly increase urinary citrate and be beneficial in reducing recurrent stones. Finally, an over-the-counter product you can buy on Amazon called Moonstone increases urinary citrate and has been shown to be beneficial. But beware, many supplements being promoted in the media and on the internet claim to prevent recurrent stone formation. They don't.

Another dietary factor that increases the risk of stones forming is a diet high in animal protein. Throughout my practice of over thirty years, few vegetarians or vegans came to me with stones, which should tell you something about calcium oxalate stone prevention. Diets high in grains, nuts, seeds, legumes, and tuberous vegetables further decrease the risk. There is evidence that in older adults, magnesium, potassium and increased fluid intake reduced risk, whereas intake of Vitamin C increased the risk.

The next thing you'll want to do is limit your salt (sodium or Na+) intake. Salt is everywhere and in everything, so check labels. Processed foods, takeout foods, and any food served in a restaurant tends to be high in salt. Replace salt with spices and/or lemon for flavor. Excretion of Na+ and calcium are linked, so by restricting salt, you will decrease the amount of calcium in the urine.

Some patients assume limiting the amount of calcium and calcium containing foods in their diet prevents new stone formation. It's rational to think limiting dietary calcium will decrease the amount of calcium in the urine, and thus prevent more stones from forming. As it turns out, however, the concentration of oxalate in the urine is a more important determinant of recurrent stone formation than the concentration of calcium. A lot of **dietary oxalate results in increased oxalate concentration in the urine, which, behind hydration, salt, and protein, is the fourth most important factor in recurrent ca-ox stones.**

Calcium oxalate is a salt. If you ingest enough calcium, that calcium binds to oxalate in the gut and prevents GI absorption of some of the oxalate. The calcium oxalate in the gut gets absorbed a lot less from the gut than free oxalate, so you poop oxalate bound to calcium out. It stands to reason then that it's more important to reduce dietary oxalate, than it is to restrict calcium. In fact, we don't want you to restrict dietary calcium at all.

Prevention of Calcium Oxalate Stones

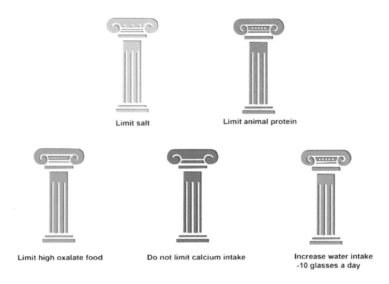

5 pillars of calcium oxalate stone prevention

But we do want you to watch your oxalate intake. Foods high in oxalate include spinach and other leafy green vegetables, soy, almonds, potatoes, beets, navy beans, raspberries, and more. This is one time that I'd recommend Googling "foods high in oxalate" and see if you are ingesting one of the many culprit foods high in oxalate. Some of these foods high in oxalate have health benefit, so I'm not saying eliminate them entirely, just limit it. A low oxalate diet combined with proper hydration is preferable. I recently had a friend who endured a three month ordeal with a calcium oxalate stone. After it was resolved we talked about his diet to which he replied, "my wife and I eat spinach almost every night."

In short, I would instruct my patients on the "five pillars" for reducing calcium oxalate stones—drink a lot of water throughout the day, limit salt intake, eat minimal animal protein (which includes dairy products, especially ones high in animal fat such as butter and cream), watch your dietary oxalate, and don't decrease your calcium intake.

Because diet and hydration are so important in stone disease, I had all of my patients (first timers *and* frequent flyers with recurrent stones) keep a diet diary for two weeks. I'd request that they write everything down, the time of day that they ate or drank, pills/medication, and the amount. From the diary I'd get an idea of their hydration habits, and I'd be able to see if there was anything in the diet to cause stone formation.

What about cranberry juice? Most people assume that cranberry juice is good for your kidneys and urinary tract. This is true if you are prone to urinary tract infections, but it's not true if you've had calcium oxalate stones, because cranberry juice has a lot of oxalate in it. Similarly, grapefruit juice has also been associated with a high risk of stone formation.

Large amounts of vitamin C will cause calcium oxalate stones to form, so you don't want to take vitamin C supplements. Most people get enough vitamin C in the diet, so there is no need to take extra. Besides, large amounts of vitamin C has never been shown to prevent colds or make colds go away faster, despite the myths that they do.

We've just been talking about first time calcium oxalate stone formers. If this is your second time around with a calcium oxalate stone, or if the stone analysis shows a stone type other than calcium oxalate, the evaluation becomes a little more involved. No matter what kind of stone you have, the goal is to keep you stone free, we'll want to dig a deeper and do what's called a "metabolic work up" in addition to the standard history, physical exam, blood tests and diet diary. A metabolic work up is basically collecting urine over 24 hours and measuring important chemicals and compounds within the urine - pH or the amount of acid in urine, sodium, potassium, chloride, citrate, oxalate, calcium, uric acid, and creatinine.

Putting all the variables together will help us decide if you could benefit from more treatment in addition to the five pillars of prevention. A metabolic work-up can be done by a urologist specializing in stones, or it can be done by a primary care provider with an interest and expertise in stone prevention, or it can be done by an endocrinologist. There are additional medications that may be beneficial if you are a recurrent stone former. And there are several promising therapies (probiotics, gene modification) on the horizon.

Bladder Stones

Bladder stones are more common in men over 50 because they form in stagnant urine. If you've read the chapter on BPH you'll understand that an enlarged prostate is the most common (but not the only cause) of urine that doesn't get peed out. Urine that stays in the bladder allows the crystals to get together and form a stone. Stones can also occur in an out-pouching in the bladder called a "diverticulum" (an abnormal sac or out pouching). They also form in both men and women who don't empty their bladders because of nerve damage (diabetes, spinal cord injury, or multiple sclerosis for example). Bladder stones can be single or multiple and range in size from the size of a pencil eraser to a tennis ball. They are frequently associated with a urinary tract infection. Most bladder stones are treated through the urethra using lasers, ultrasound, or an instrument I favored called a "litho-clast" (combination of ultrasound and pneumatic energy). It's important to not only remove the stone but treat the cause of the stagnant urine.

Conclusion

If you've made it this far, this may be your first journey through stone hell, or you may have been there before, maybe more than once. As you know, having a stone can be a dreadful experience, and you are faced with many decisions: should I wait and see if the stone passes, or should I go for a procedure to remove it? If I chose to have a procedure, should I agree to have the one that will get rid of it, or should I opt for a less invasive procedure that may leave residual fragments which could require another procedure? What caused my stone(s) and what can I do to keep them from coming back? If you are currently plagued with a stone sitting somewhere in your urinary tract, you'll want to work with your urologist to make a shared decision about what to do about it. You have options, and the options should be explained to you with respect to risks and benefits of each potential procedure. We have many tools in the toolbox to help you through this hellish experience, and rest assured, these tools (lasers, ESWL, ultrasonic lithotripsy) have made modern day treatment of stones much better than it was 30 or 40 years ago. "Cutting for stone" very rarely happens these days. Once the acute episode is resolved, hopefully you can now appreciate how critical hydration and other dietary measures are for prevention. Together you and your urologist will get you out of a painful experience you never want to have again.

CHAPTER 11

Kidney Tumors, Cysts, and Masses

This is a chapter you probably won't be reading unless you or a loved one have, or may have, a tumor or mass in the kidney. Our lives depend on having at least one functioning kidney, yet those of us with healthy kidneys don't think about them all that much. It's only when something goes wrong that we turn our attention to these life supporting organs. Finding a tumor or mass in a kidney is a discovery that gets our attention.

Any tumor or mass in the kidney is cause for concern because it could be cancer. The most common type of kidney cancer is renal cell carcinoma, or RCC. In the United States there will be 73,000 new cases of RCC each year, and 15,000 will die each year. Though anyone can get it, it is more common in men, African Americans, and Native Americans. RCC is an aggressive cancer with a survival rate of 35%, which is a discouraging statistic if you receive the diagnosis. Fortunately, there have been significant advances in treatment of renal cell carcinoma of all stages. For localized kidney cancers, those that have not spread outside of the kidney, laparoscopic and robotic assisted laparoscopic removal of either part or all of the kidney have become the norm, which represents a major advance in caring for kidney cancer patients over the past 15 years.

RFA (radiofrequency ablation) and cryoablation (freezing) are good options in certain circumstances, and result in decent cancer control and survival for some patients who may not be able to tolerate a more involved operation. Finally, there have been significant advances with a wide variety of chemotherapeutic agents over the past 15 years. There are also ongoing clinical trials that are studying new "targeted" therapy. Survival rates are improving, and should continue to improve, though metastatic kidney cancer is still a very serious condition. So what does it mean for you if you receive the news that a tumor or mass has been detected in one or both kidneys? Let's consider the possibilities.

Renal Masses

A renal mass is a general term for any abnormal growth in the kidney. Renal masses can be benign or malignant, they can be single or multiple, they may or may not cause pain, they may or may not produce blood in the urine, and they vary in size from a half inch to over ten or more inches and can affect all or just a portion of the kidney. Renal masses are often discovered by chance, when doctors are looking for something else, and turn up on an ultrasound, CT scan, or MRI. However they are discovered and whatever their state, the first thing your urologist will want to determine is if the mass is solid or cystic.

A cystic mass is one that is filled with fluid. The fluid can be a water-like protein or it may be blood (a "hemorrhagic cyst"). Most renal cysts do not produce symptoms, but depending on the type of renal cyst, it may or may not be malignant. How do you know which type of cyst you have? Your urologist will want you to have diagnostic imaging tests, which will be reviewed by a radiologist and your urologist who will use a series of objective criteria to determine certain characteristics of the cyst. CT scans done for renal lesions, both cystic and solid, are first done prior to the administration of intravenous contrast. After the non-contrast CT, an IV contrast is injected (which shouldn't cause any pain or discomfort) and the scan is repeated. Renal cysts that have the potential of being malignant will take up the contrast and "light up" or show what's called "contrast enhancement." Those that are benign will not enhance or take up contrast.

Once imaging (usually CT but can also be ultrasound and/or MRI) is completed the results are reviewed. Kidney cysts are classified according to something called the Bosniak classification system, which classifies them as I, II, II-F, III, and IV. A Bosniak I cyst is a simple kidney cyst. These B-I cysts usually do not cause any symptoms unless they become so large that they press upon the surrounding organs, which is rare. B-I cysts are quite common (nearly half of people over 50 have them) and do not need to be treated in any way.

A cyst that meets true Bosniak II classification is also benign and does not need treatment. B-II cysts are slightly more complicated on the CT. There can be separations within the cyst, and these thin walls that traverse the cyst are usually not calcified. B-II-F cysts are slightly more complicated, however. A B-IIF cyst can have more septa and calcifications, but do not take up contrast or enhance. The "F" stands for "Follow" because even though 75 to 95% of these cysts are benign, some will take on the radiographic appearance of a more ominous cyst later. For that reason, urologists recommend yearly ultrasounds or CT scans to be sure they aren't growing or changing in any way, or in other words, not changing from benign to malignant.[xiii]

Bosniak III cysts are characterized by multiple septa of varying thickness and can have varying amounts of calcification within them. Fifty percent of B-III cysts are malignant and therefore it's generally recommended that they be removed. A biopsy of B-III cysts is not recommended, because it's easy to miss cancer if present. There are several surgical options for removing the mass including laparoscopic or open surgery. If the location of the mass allows removal of the mass with a "margin" of normal kidney, this is called a "partial nephrectomy." Sometimes, however, a B-III cyst is in the central portion of the kidney and partial removal is not possible because it would either jeopardize the collecting system of the blood vessels that supply or drain blood from the kidney. The bottom line is that no matter the size of the cyst, if it's a B-III, it should be removed.

B-IV cysts are malignant and these, too, need to be removed either by partial or total nephrectomy.

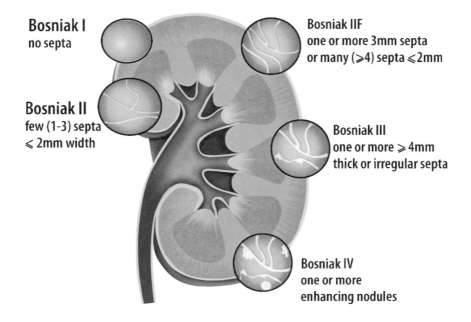

Bosniak I
no septa

Bosniak II
few (1-3) septa
≤ 2mm width

Bosniak IIF
one or more 3mm septa
or many (≥4) septa ≤2mm

Bosniak III
one or more ≥ 4mm
thick or irregular septa

Bosniak IV
one or more
enhancing nodules

Bosniak Classification system of kidney cysts

Before we move on to solid renal masses, a few more words about renal cysts. Although rare, cysts can become infected. If this happens, you will usually have flank pain (pain in your upper abdomen, back or sides), fever, and an elevated white blood cell count. A cyst can also rupture, but this is also rare. Cyst rupture is characterized by sudden and sometimes severe flank pain. And a cyst can become so large that is blocks the outflow of urine from the kidney or can press on surrounding organs and cause pain. All three of these conditions are rare, however, so if you are diagnosed with a benign cyst, it's unlikely to cause you any problems.

There is an inherited condition called Adult Polycystic Kidney Disease (APKD). The inheritance pattern can be either autosomal dominant or recessive. If you have APKD, there can be hundreds of cysts in each kidney and the kidneys can be so large that they cause abdominal or flank pain. Sometimes there are so many cysts that they replace the entire functioning tissue of the kidney, which results in renal failure. People with APKD are prone to hypertension. There is an increased association with aneurisms (balloon dilation of blood vessels). Patients with APKD can also have multiple cysts in their liver. Patients with huge kidneys due to APKD can have severe bothersome symptoms (abdominal distention, pain, bloating, nausea and vomiting), simply due to the size of the kidneys. In these cases, it's sometimes necessary to surgically puncture all the cysts to make room for the other abdominal organs. Also, when APKD leads to renal failure, there are times when both non-functioning kidneys are removed before renal transplantation.

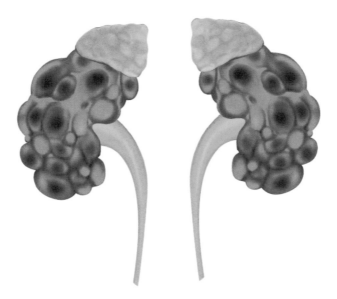

Adult Polysysistic Kidney Disease

What if the mass is solid? That's when you're likely wondering, is it cancer? Am I going to die? Well, that depends. The size of the tumor matters. Age matters. Co-morbid conditions matter. What the mass looks like under the microscope matters.

The smaller the renal mass, the more likely it is going to be benign. What is small? Well, let's say "small" is less than 0.5 inch or a centimeter. Solid renal tumors are that size or less are usually benign. The bigger the mass, however, the more likely it is to be malignant. Yet not all large renal masses (more than half an inch or 1.0 cm) are malignant. Of those that are malignant, about 90% are going to be "renal cell carcinoma" or "adenocarcinoma of the kidney" or "clear cell carcinoma of the kidney." These three names all describe the same cancer, renal cell cancer, what we call RCC or RCCa. As far as your urologist is concerned, all solid renal tumors should be considered RCCa (renal cell cancer) until proven otherwise, even the small ones. So what happens if a solid mass is found?

If you are found to have a solid renal mass, the size and radiologic features (CT/MRI) will point toward it being malignant. Before embarking on treatment, your urologist will want to know if the cancer has spread to other parts of your body. This is called a metastatic work-up. Since kidney cancer is one of the more common cancers to spread to bone, your urologist will order a bone scan and several blood tests. One of the blood tests is called alkaline phosphatase and can be elevated in the presence of bone metastases. Kidney cancer also spreads to lymph nodes in the retroperitoneum, abdomen, chest, and anywhere else in the body where there are lymph nodes. For that reason, a CT scans of the chest is done. You will have already had a CT or MRI of the abdomen and pelvis.

Whether or not to biopsy the tumor is a matter of controversy. Some urologists feel that there's no harm in doing a biopsy. But it can be easy to miss RCCa on biopsy, and imaging tests are pretty good in determining whether it's malignant. A biopsy may be indicated if we can't tell whether the mass is benign or malignant based on CT or MRI. My view is that the urologist should ask whether or not a biopsy will affect the treatment they are likely to recommend. For example, a 3.0 cm (golf ball size) solid mass in a 75 year old with multiple medical problems would likely be managed by active surveillance, even if it does enhance on CT/MRI, so the results of a biopsy, whether benign or malignant, would not alter what I'd recommend to my patient, so I would not advise a biopsy. Or say the patient is 50 and has a 5 cm (2 inch) tumor that enhances on CT/MRI and has no fat in it (fat appears as black on imaging, and usually means its benign tumor called an angiomyolipoma). A renal tumor that enhances and has no fat in it is most likely cancer. Removal needs to be done regardless, so why risk a biopsy when it's not going to change what we'd recommend? Or consider my friend's 86 year old mother, who was suffering from dementia when a solid mass was found on her right kidney. She most likely had a malignancy. However, because of her age and other medical problems, she would not benefit from having surgery, so even if the biopsy proved that it was malignant, we would not recommend that it be removed. If the patient were younger, however, and we couldn't tell by imaging if the mass was benign or malignant, a biopsy could be in order because if it showed benign tissue, the patient could avoid having unnecessary surgery.

A biopsy of a renal mass should be considered when the results will change what you would do about it. There are cases when the radiologist and urologist will be unable to tell if the mass is malignant or benign. There are other solid masses of the kidney that are not benign, but they aren't primary kidney tumors, which means they didn't originate in the kidney. For example, non-renal cancers that are found in the kidney are lymphomas or metastatic(s) lesions from a non-renal source. In the case of lymphoma, chemotherapy, not surgery, is usually the first and best treatment option. Certain infectious processes can also look like renal masses, and these problems are usually treated with antibiotics (unless in the case of an abscess that requires surgical drainage.

Stage and Grade

Let's assume you are anxiously awaiting the results of your testing when your urologist breaks the bad news: you have kidney cancer. What's next? Your treatment will depend upon the stage and grade of your cancer. How are cancer stage and grade determined, and why are they important? Stage refers to the size and extent of the cancer, and grade refers to what the cancer looks like under the microscope—the appearance of the cells and the architecture of how the cells are arranged. The more abnormal the individual cells appear and the more abnormal the architecture, the higher the grade.

The staging system most often used for most cancers including kidney, prostate, and bladder cancer worldwide is the **TNM** system, discussed in Chapter 7. Recall that the "T" stands for tumor and refers to the size of the mass, how much of the organ (in this case the kidney) the tumor occupies, whether it has grown into critical structures within the kidney, if it's grown beyond the boundary of the outer kidney capsule into the surrounding fat, and if it had grown into surrounding organs. A number 1-4 is assigned to the T stage, the lower the number, the better.

The spread to lymph nodes is signified by "N." Your urologist will want to know if the cancer spread to nearby lymph nodes or distant lymph nodes. The N "number" varies according to which lymph nodes are positive (adjacent to the kidney, or distant), how many nodes appear positive, and the size of the positive nodes. If surgery hasn't been done yet, the N number is assessed by imaging (CT, MRI, or PET). If nodes are removed at the same time the kidney cancer is removed, and they have cancer in them. Your surgeon and pathologist will determine the "N" number, based on what they find.

The "M" stands for metastasis. Renal cell carcinoma spreads to other parts of the body by getting into the blood or lymphatic vessels. RCC has an affinity for spreading to bone and lung, and rarely to brain, liver, adrenal gland, and pancreas. If you have metastatic disease, your urologist and radiation oncologist will work with your urologist to determine the best course of action. There are circumstances in which a person may have metastatic disease and depending on the number and location of the cancer, all three treatment modalities (radiation, chemo, and surgery) may be your best option. There are other circumstances in which surgery will be of no benefit, and it would be best to treat you with chemo alone.

The TNM assigned to each kidney cancer is determined before surgery. This is the "clinical" stage and is based on physical exam, possible biopsies (tumor, lymph nodes, bone), and imaging tests (CT,

MRI, bone and PET scans). If surgery is done, the "pathologic" stage is determined by examining tissue (the tumor itself, possibly the entire kidney with the tumor in it if the whole thing is removed, and possibly lymph nodes if a node dissection is done). This cancer staging may be complex and confusing so if you have any questions about your TNM stage, please ask your doctor to explain it to you in a way you understand. Along with tumor grade, the stage is important in what treatment options are best for your particular situation.

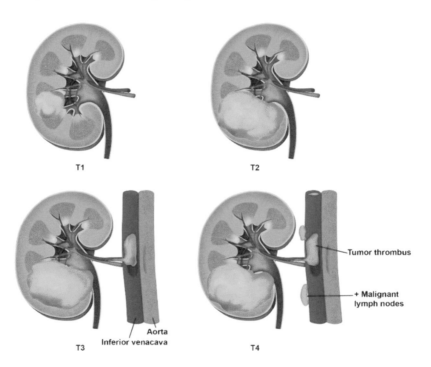

Stages of kidney cancer – renal cell carcinoma

In addition to stage and grade, your age, general health status, and any existing co-morbidities, also play a role in deciding which treatment options are best. For cancers confined to the kidney (T1 and T2), laparoscopic and robotic assisted laparoscopic removal of either part or all of the kidney have become the norm. Radiofrequency ablation (RFA) and cryoablation (freezing) are good options in certain circumstances, and result in decent cancer control and survival for some patients who may not be able to tolerate a more involved operation.

There have also been significant advances with a wide variety of chemotherapeutic agents over the past 15 years. There are ongoing clinical trials that are studying new "targeted" therapy. Survival rates are improving, and should continue to improve, though metastatic kidney cancer is still a very serious condition. If you are unfortunate to have Stage IV metastatic renal cell carcinoma, you will best be served by an oncologist who is familiar with the variety of newer chemotherapy strategies, and the ongoing clinical trials that employ these new drugs.

Conclusion

In summary, if you are seeing a urologist for a kidney tumor, you'll want to know if it's cystic or solid, benign or malignant. If your urologist can't tell, you'll want to be aware of how you can find out using various imaging techniques, and possibly having the mass biopsied. If your urologist says it's most likely benign, you'll want to know what you need to do to follow it to be sure it stays benign, that is, will it grow or change into something that's malignant? Some benign kidney tumors (angiomyolipoma, for example), can grow larger. As these benign tumors increase in size (bigger than a plum or 4.5 cm) the more likely they are to bleed, which can be catastrophic.

If the mass is likely malignant, you'll also want to participate in a Shared Decision Making discussion with your urologist and learn about the various options for treatment, the risks and potential benefits of each treatment option, and the differences in the 5, 10, and 15 year survival. Don't hesitate to write your questions down. "If I have just the part of the kidney with the tumor in it removed, or removal just the tumor, as opposed to removing all the kidney and tumor, is there a difference in survival?" "What are the potential complications of a robotic assisted lap nephrectomy (kidney removal using laparoscopes and the robot)? How are they different from an open nephrectomy? What's the difference in how many days I'll be in the hospital? What's the difference in recovery time, when will I be able to play pickleball again?" "Would I benefit from having chemo before you take my kidney tumor out?" "Do I need to see an oncologist? Radiation oncologist?" "What would happen if I don't have surgery?" And more.

Yes, there are lots of questions. I'll frequently get a call from a friend, relative, or friend of a friend saying "They say I have a kidney tumor and that it might be cancer. What should I ask the urologist?" I hope that this chapter will help answer your questions. Ideally your urologist will have the time to go through all your options so that you and they can arrive at the best decision.

CHAPTER 12

Erectile Dysfunction

When people find out that I'm a urologist, I get asked a lot of questions, and I hear a lot of stories about previous encounters with urologists. Whether it's prostate issues, problems peeing, kidney stones, infections, blood in the urine, scrotal issues, or cancers, there isn't a topic on urology that someone hasn't asked me about outside the office—except for one. The one area that I never get asked about is impotence or sexual/erectile dysfunction. Never. Not once outside of my office. I guess as long as I wore a white coat and was seeing people in a professional capacity, impotence was an acceptable topic to discuss. But outside the clinic, ED was taboo. So here are some answers to some questions you may have been afraid to ask.

Originally, I didn't feel the need to write a chapter on impotence. I thought, heck, any guy having trouble getting it up can go online and get Viagra, why do I need to even discuss it? In fact, while writing this chapter I have the Cardinal-Red Sox game on in the background. They are in between innings and there is a commercial blaring for some online pharmacy which is urging viewers to, "Order your Viagra now, no prescription necessary, no doctor office visit required. And, as an added bonus, we'll provide you with testosterone support." A picture of a vial of what I assume is testosterone accompanies the urgent message to spend money now. I cringe. This kind of stuff can be dangerous to your health.

This pseudo-medical messaging is potentially dangerous, maybe even life threatening. Why? Because you want to know what the cause of the impotence is. It may be something simple, correctable, and reversible. You may not need a drug that has potential side effects. Despite the "warnings" you may hear on television for taking drugs like Viagra called PDE5 inhibitors (PDE5 stands for phosphodiesterase—Levitra and Cialis are among other commonly available PDE5 inhibitors), I would venture to guess that most men are desperate for a fix and ignore the warnings about side effects—and depending on any underlying health conditions that you may or may not know about, you might be at heightened risk for these side effects. Another reason to see a physician before taking any pill to fix your problem, is that the doctor will want to rule out possible problems that could be responsible for the ED, which could include heart disease, diabetes, neurological impairment or a vascular blockage. So feel free to order Viagra or one of its cousins off the internet without seeing a doctor, but please understand that you are taking more risks than you need to—you are risking that you don't have an underlying condition that's causing your erectile dysfunction, you are risking that there aren't better and less risky alternative treatments that may fit your needs better, and you are risking the side effects of the pill that you get off the internet (which can include heart failure, heart attack, and stroke).

Before getting into how urologists approach the problem of ED, and what you can expect on your first visit prior to taking any medication, I offer an anecdote. From 1997 to 2011 I coached competitive girls' soccer with my good friend Nick. Nick and I coached five different teams that traveled all over the country. The girls ranged in age from 12-15. One weekend we were playing in a tournament in Bellingham, Washington and found ourselves hanging around in the hotel lobby in between games when a commercial for Cialis came on. At the end of the commercial there was a warning — "Cialis can result in a prolonged erection lasting more than four hours. If this happens seek immediate medical attention!" Fifteen 13 year old girls, the other coach, and a few parents all looked at me, and unlike most adult men, they did not hesitate to ask a slew of questions.

"Eeeww, coach, does that really happen?" "What happens after four hours??" "Why does that happen?" "Does in hurt?" "Is it permanent?" "Yuck, Yuck, and more Yucks."

"Girls," I said, laughing, "Let's think about soccer and I'll answer your questions in another ten years."

Fortunately, it's been over ten years since that offer and none have returned with their questions!

Let's get something straight (no pun intended) before diving into a discussion about impotence. "Impotence" may mean different things to different people. I prefer to talk about sexual dysfunction as sexual performance and capabilities outside of what's considered normal. Erectile dysfunction is different. *Erectile dysfunction is the inability to obtain or maintain an erection.* Premature ejaculation, a common problem that affects 1 in 4 men, is not erectile dysfunction. Premature ejaculation is when a man obtains orgasm and ejaculates before their partner desires it, normally with a minute of penetration. Losing an erection prior to ejaculation and orgasm, however, a term we call "premature detumescence," is considered a form of erectile dysfunction.

A bend or curvature in an erect penis caused by scar tissue and sometimes painful is a condition called Peyronies Disease. Peyronies Disease typically does not cause erectile dysfunction, except in rare and severe cases. Nonetheless, the pain from Peyronies Disease can result in poor or undesirable erections.

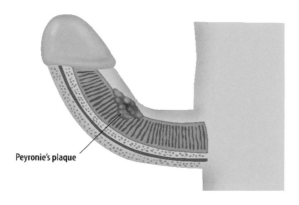

Peyronie's plaque

Peyronie's Disease

Finally, an inability to have an orgasm and or ejaculate falls under the category of sexual dysfunction but is not erectile dysfunction.

With these caveats in mind, this chapter will discuss normal erectile physiology, what can cause it to go wrong, and the many treatment options available to fix it.

A good history of the problem is a good start to figure out what's gone haywire. The first series of questions that I would ask are, "How long has this been going on? Does it happen all the time? Does your penis ever get hard? Partially? Never?" And the most important question, "Do you wake up with a normal erection, or do you know if you get erections during sleep?" These questions can give the first clue as to whether the problem is psychological or emotional verses physical. Your brain, subconscious mind, and emotions can significantly influence your erections. If you only experience the problem occasionally, and if you have normal erections when you wake up in the morning or during sleep, then the problem is most likely psychological. We call this psychogenic impotence.

Some men don't know if they get erections during sleep. Some men may wake up with "half hard piss hard-ons." When I was a junior resident, a couple the senior residents invented what they called "the stamp test." They took ordinary postage stamps and had patients who couldn't tell if they got erections during sleep to put a ring of stamps around the base of their penises before they went to sleep. If the patient got an erection during sleep, the ring would be broken in the morning. I have no idea how they thought that up, but the "penile stamp test" made Wikipedia, (though my resident buddies get no credit). What they had devised was a test for "nocturnal (night) penile tumescence (swollen in response to sexual stimulation). Since then, medical device companies have come up with fancy and expensive rings that fit around the base of the penis during sleep and are attached to an electronic monitor that measures tumescence, kind of like a blood pressure cuff for the penis, but as far as I know, they're no more accurate than the stamps, but cost from four to five thousand dollars![xiv]

For a man to have normal erections, there are several requirements—plumbing (blood flow), electricity (a normal intact nervous system from the brain down along the spinal cord through peripheral nerves to the penis and then back again in reverse order), and fuel (male hormone testosterone). All three must function normally. And at the same time, the brain, conscious, sub-conscious, and unconscious, rules over all three. This is why when you remove the conscious brain during sleep, normal or nocturnal erections occur, because the three factors are released from the mind's influence.

With organic erectile dysfunction there is something wrong with the plumbing (an example would be poor blood flow to the penis or the valves that hold blood in during erection don't work properly resulting in premature detumescence), electricity (the nerves going to the penis are damaged or cut during prostate surgery), or there isn't enough fuel (low male hormone testosterone). When this happens many men get depressed, anxious, or both, and then we have a psychological problem on top of a physical or organic one.

For many reasons, I don't think that the "internet doctor" solution for ordering Viagra is always a good one. If you have psychogenic impotence and everything else checks out and you get erections in your sleep or when you wake up in the morning, you may not want to take a pill that can have significant side effects. You may not need any medication at all.

For men with psychogenic impotence, I recommend they address the problem by starting with a book called *The New Male Sexuality* by Bernie Zilbergeld. I read the book when I was a resident and have been recommending it to patients with erectile dysfunction ever since as it's become a classic. Within the book are clear explanations for why some men suffer from all forms of ED. There are suggested exercises in the book that have proven helpful. Most importantly, you should read the book with your partner. As a cooperative team you may be able to fix the issue without medication. Even if you don't have a cooperative partner, I'd still get the book, and then I'd seek couples counseling or sexual counseling. Your therapist may still recommend a PDE5 inhibitor like Viagra. Or the therapist may think that another drug to treat depression or anxiety would be best.

If you have organic impotence, however, I'd still recommend that you *not* get Viagra off the internet without first seeing your primary care provider. Your penis is like a canary in a coal mine. That is, your ED may be the first sign of a more serious problem. Your primary care provider will do a history (including a sexual and psychosocial history) and physical. Lab tests will be ordered in an effort to find out what's killing the canary. S/he will ask you about your heart and circulation, do a vascular exam (feel your pulses), check your nervous system, and do blood tests for diabetes for example, cholesterol and lipids, and male hormone levels (since testosterone levels vary during the day it's best to do the blood draw in the morning). If your sex drive is low, s/he may also order a hormone blood test called prolactin.

If your PCP discovers something that could be contributing to your ED s/he may treat it without referring you to a urologist. An example would be if your male hormone level is very low, your doctor would likely investigate why it's low. Say you had mumps as a kid and it affected your testicles and they aren't making enough testosterone, you could start treatment for your ED not by taking Viagra but by taking testosterone which comes in many forms (a dermal patch, injections, and pills). I've found that injections work best.

The goal of therapy is to return male hormone levels to the normal range, and not exceed the upper limit of normal. You need to be aware of the risks associated with testosterone therapy to include heart attack, stroke, acne, and mood swings. Testosterone causes growth of prostate cancer, and benign prostate cells, as well as breast cancer. Normally testosterone levels go down as we get older, but if you're elderly with low normal testosterone I'd advise against treatment with testosterone replacement therapy because the cardiovascular risks and effect testosterone has on the prostate are too great. Sometimes treatment can be as simple as a change in diet, or may require quitting smoking, alcohol or other drugs that can cause ED (marijuana is a good example).

What can you expect when you see a urologist? Like your PCP, your urologist will first try to differentiate whether your ED is psychogenic or organic. We've discussed an approach to psychogenic impotence, and let's assume your testosterone is normal. The urologist will repeat the history and physical looking for clues. S/he will look over your lab results, which hopefully will include a PSA. Once they've made a diagnosis, it's then time for a shared decision making conversation regarding the risks and benefits of the many available treatment options.

What I'm going to say now applies to all men suffering from organic impotence regardless of cause. That includes men with ED after prostate cancer surgery. All forms of therapy should be discussed because some will work better than others. It's also true that the risks differ among the various options. One form of therapy may be more suited for one man, while not suited for another, depending on the cause of the ED, though there are times when the culprit is not known. The benefit of shared decision making is that the doctor considers all these variables and will want to tailor therapy to your lifestyle, personal preferences, and how much risk you want to take. For example, Viagra might not be the best medication for you because you may have heart disease, but if you don't want to have surgery (penile prosthesis), there are still several other options. Let's discuss the risk and benefits of these options so can make the best decision for therapy for you.

TestosteroneThe "fuel" needed for an erection is your male hormone, testosterone. As we've discussed, your doctor will measure your testosterone, but there are other hints that your testosterone may be low such as a loss of sexual desire or libido, easy fatigue, weakness and loss of muscle mass, and inability to focus or concentrate. Other physical signs of low T are weak bones, obesity despite dieting and exercising, and a predisposition to diabetes and high bad cholesterol (LDL).

Replacing the testosterone you need is not just for sex, but for many aspects of your overall health. Usually, testosterone is measured in the morning, and before a definite diagnosis of low testosterone is made, several measurements are required, along with the measurement of certain proteins that are attached to some of the testosterone molecules. This is what doctors are talking about when they say "free" testosterone (testosterone that is not bound to protein). Low testosterone conditions are reversible and some can be improved by dietary modification. But most low testosterone conditions are permanent. If your testosterone is low, your doctor will try to determine why it's low, and whether the low T is reversible, or not. Many internists and family practice providers can help you with this without a urology referral.

Endocrinologists are skilled at finding out why me have low testosterone levels and treating it.

If your testosterone is low, please do not try to replace it yourself without the knowledge and expertise of a doctor, such as an internist, family practitioner, urologist, or endocrinologist. You want to know that you are being treated with the appropriate dose administered in the most effective way, whether that's oral pills, shots, gels, implants, or nasal sprays. Also, you want someone monitoring you for dangerous side effects. Be careful because there's a lot of stuff out there claiming to boost your testosterone "naturally" when there is actually real testosterone in the pill.

Before treating anyone for low testosterone it's important to know that they don't have prostate cancer because if cancer is present, testosterone is like adding gasoline to a fire and will stimulate the cancer to grow and possibly spread. Some urologists have been taught not to give testosterone to any man who has had a history of prostate cancer, but if the prostate cancer has been cured (zero PSA after a prostatectomy), most think it's fine to do testosterone replacement.

Too much testosterone can cause problems with your liver, skin, and cause an abnormal increase in your red blood cells, a condition called polycythemia. The goal of testosterone replacement therapy should be to get testosterone levels to the 400 - 600 range. Any more than 600 does you no good and puts you at risk for more dangerous side effects. Beside hopefully restoring your sexual function, normal testosterone has benefits for your overall health, mood, ability to focus and concentrate, and exercise. The bottom line, though, is that if your testosterone is low, the benefits to replacement therapy outweigh the risks, but only when done under the care of a knowledgeable health care provider.

Okay, so your testosterone is normal, and you finally say, "Just give me the blue pill doc." Not so fast. Though Viagra and the other PDE5 inhibitors will "fix" many organic and psychogenic ED problems, the little blue pill may not be the best alternative, since there can be side effects from the medication, or the medication may not work, or maybe you just don't want to take another pill. So before discussing Viagra and the other PDE5 inhibitors, let's discuss other alternative treatments.

Vacuum Erection Devices

A vacuum erection device (also known as a penis pump) does not require a prescription and you won't need any medication. The device consists of a clear cylinder that is placed over the penis and held tight against the pubis to create a seal. The device is then attached via a tube to either a mechanical pump or a battery charged pump that creates a vacuum inside the cylinder. This vacuum causes a filling of the erectile tissue with blood, which is really all an erection is anyway. Once the penis is erect, a silicone rubber band, which had been placed on the pubic end of the cylinder, is slid off the device and onto the base of the penis (google "cock ring" if you need to know more). The rubber band holds the blood in the erect penis until the fun is over. It won't make the penis any larger than it was before and since almost half of the erectile tissue is underneath the pubic bone and not subject to the pressure the vacuum creates, that part of the penis on the body side of the band will not get hard. Consequently, some men complain that the penis is like a "hinge" but all in all, it does the trick.

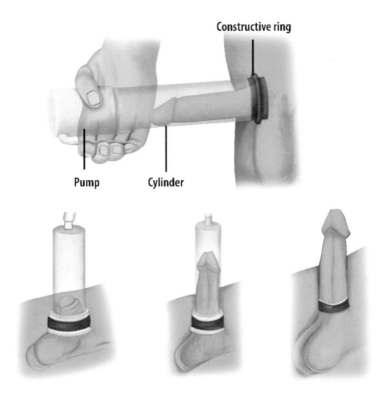

Vacuum Erection Device for ED

The VED has other benefits. If the ED is a result of poor blood flow, over time the erectile tissue is starved of blood and oxygen. When tissue doesn't get enough oxygen it will die off and be replaced by scar tissue. By bringing fresh oxygenated blood into the penis a VED can improve the health of the erectile tissue. The same phenomena occurs if the ED is a result of prostate surgery for cancer. Think of it as a "rehab device" for your penis. The VED can be used in combination with other treatments, and it can be reused. I've seen very few complications with the VED. Of the few complaints I've heard, most have been mild bruising, which of course can be worse if you're on blood thinners, but for most men it's a quick and easy solution.

Alternative Medications

I was in practice one year in 1983 attending the annual American Urologic Meeting in Las Vegas. I was attending meetings all day (and keeping my eye on the black jack table) when I heard a loud commotion down the hall from one of the meeting rooms. Several minutes later the room emptied of all these esteemed urologists, and their wives, who had been attending a dinner meeting.

My ex-boss and Urology Department Chair at OHSU (Dr John Barry) walked by. "What happened in there, Dr Barry?" I asked him.

"You would not believe it Lieberman," he answered, shaking his head.

"Try me."

"This crazy British physiologist just dropped his pants in front of everyone to demonstrate an erection that he produced by injecting his penis with phentolamine. It caused quite a stir." (Remember, this was 15 years before Viagra was accidentally discovered in 1998.)

As you can imagine that presentation was the only thing anyone was talking about that year!

But humor aside, his demonstration points to the fact that Viagra and other PDE5 inhibitors are not the only medications available for ED. Due to the many side effects and the potential for complications if there are underlying health issues, the little blue pill is not the answer for about one third of men with organic ED. If you're among that third, what else might you consider? There are several other medications that can be injected directly into the erectile tissue (prostaglandin, papaverine, and phentolamine) that will produce an erection in most men. Prostaglandin also comes as a urethral suppository called alprostadil. This preparation is a small pellet about the size of a grain of rice that is inserted into the urethra. The other three drugs are combined in an injectable preparation called "Triple P."

Currently intracorporal injections are commonly done with a combination of the three medications as a preparation called TriMix. This treatment is 90% effective. Our pharmacy made up the prep we called "Triple P." Because the drugs are injected locally, there are few side effects. A worrisome thing that can occur is priapism, which is a prolonged erection that lasts more than a few hours. Then there are local risks associated with putting a needle into the penis such as bruising and infection. If you and your urologist decide on intracorporal injections, you'll need to learn the proper technique for administering the medication to limit the side effects.

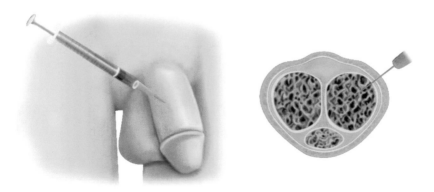

Intracorporal Injection Therapy for ED

Viagra

Viagra hit the market in 1998 after it was discovered that men taking it for cardiac problems were getting erections. What a fortuitous discovery! Like its cousins Levitra and Cialis, Viagra dilates the blood vessels in the erectile tissue and allows the penis to fill with blood and oxygen. It should be taken 30-60 minutes before sex. Erections typically last an hour or two depending on your metabolism, the dose, and what you had to eat or drink.

Before starting Viagra (hopefully given to you via prescription from a physician) if you are taking any medications at all, you'll want to check with your doctor regarding potential drug interactions.[xv]

Viagra also interacts with grapefruit juice. Other potential side effects include headaches, low blood pressure and/or flushing. Also, Viagra is contraindicated if you have heart disease and another long list of medical problems. Well known side effects include upset stomach, flushing, stuffy nose, and vision changes.

Surgical Implants

If all else fails, there's always surgery, as in penile implants. There are three varieties of penile prostheses. What all three have in common is that the implants are placed into each of the erectile chambers (recall from Chapter 1 that there are two erectile chambers called "corpora cavernosa"). The oldest of these implants are permanent rigid rods. The next variation is a semirigid or malleable rods, and the third is called "an inflatable," which comes as a two or three piece device. With the three piece inflatable, cylinders are attached via tubing to a pump mechanism that is placed in the scrotum. The pump in turn is connected to a reservoir of saline which is placed behind the pubic bone. When the pump is successively squeezed, saline is transferred from the reservoir into the cylinder, and the penis becomes erect. When finished, there's a button on the pump which when depressed allows the fluid to transfer back into the reservoir from the inflatable cylinders.

Penile implant surgery has been around for 40 years. Most urologists are trained to perform the surgery, which is done under local or spinal anesthesia. Complications are the same as any surgical procedure and include excessive bleeding, infection (which may require removal of the implant), injury to the urethra, bladder, or scrotal contents. Also, the implants can erode through the tough tissue that surrounds the erectile tissue. The one disadvantage of the three piece inflatable device is that it's a hydraulic system and any leak anywhere along the course of the implant will cause failure of the entire device in which case it will need to be replaced.

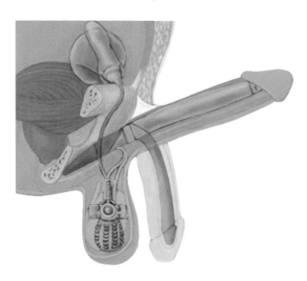

3 Piece Inflatable Penile Prosthesis

Future Innovations

There are several interesting experimental treatments for ED on the horizon that you may have heard of and include low intensity shock wave therapy, stem cells injected into the erectile tissue, and platelet rich plasma therapy. As with any experimental treatment in medicine, if you want to give any of them a try, make sure you are part of a clinical study that is testing these new therapies.

Conclusion

One of the reasons for writing this book about common urologic problems is to provide you with information necessary to make shared decisions with your physician. But sometimes the physician and patient have two different goals in mind, as my patient Floyd once taught me.

Floyd had had bladder cancer and a urethral stricture. He was in his 80s, unmarried, and living in assisted living.

To follow his bladder cancer, I needed to see him every three months, and during every visit he would say, "Doc, do you put in those penile implants?" This was before Viagra, and one of the few effective treatments for ED at the time.

"Yeah Floyd," I'd tell him, "But we need to make sure that your bladder cancer and stricture don't come back. Besides, are you even married?"

"No, she died a few years ago."

"Girlfriend?"

"Lots"

"Lots? Where are you living?"

"I live in an assisted living place."

"Well, I can offer you a VED (vacuum erection device), but no prosthesis for now. I think it's too risky."

"I don't want the penis pump, Doc, I want an implant, the kind you pump up and down."

"We'll talk about it next time," I'd say, each time.

I managed to put him off for about a year and a half. Then during one visit he came in with a "friend" who looked like he could be a starting linebacker for the Seahawks. The friend said, "Doc, you gotta put one of them implants in my buddy Floyd." He crossed his arms across his chest making it clear that he meant business.

"Well," I said, wondering what this friend was doing telling me how to treat my patient, "He's got these other problems, and…."

"No, Doc," he says, in no mood for discussion. "You don't put the implant in Floyd, we'll be calling our lawyer!"

"Okay, Okay," I said, not too happy to be bullied into a treatment I didn't recommend, but also knowing that if the patient was going to demand it, I wanted to make sure it was done right. "I'll do it, but I'm not sure it's the best option, and he's gotta understand the risks and potential complications."

"Do it Doc," the tough guy repeats, "Or the next time he'll come with his lawyer."

So I put an inflatable three-piece penile prosthesis in Floyd, and despite my reservations, he did great. No complications! No problems! Floyd was pleased as can be once I showed him how to work it, thanking me profusely.

Then, about three months after the surgery, I got a thank you note—not from Floyd, but from one of his girlfriends in the assisted living place. Her name was Sophie, and she wrote in a shaky scrawl, "Thanks you so much doctor for taking care of Floyd's problem!"

I thought that was cute and saved the letter.

A week later I received *another* thank you note. This one was from another woman named Agnes! Just as with Sophie's letter, Agnes thanked me for solving Floyd's "problem!"

I saved both thank you notes thinking that no one would believe this story.

The moral of this story is, no matter how old you are, you don't have to live with your ED, we are here to help. Better to let us help you than to try and solve the problem on your own.

CHAPTER 13

Vasectomy

Are you thinking about having a vasectomy? Perhaps you're in midlife, have children, and you definitely don't want anymore. Your wife is tired of taking birth control pills, using a diaphragm, or doesn't want to live with an IUD. Or you may have never fathered a child before, and never want to have kids for a variety of reasons and want to ensure you don't. Whatever the reason, if you are considering a vasectomy, you probably have a lot of questions.

A vasectomy is a safe and highly effective means of permanent male sterilization. In fact, vasectomies are now more commonly done than the other form of permanent female sterilization, including tubal ligation and hysterectomy.

In a general urology practice vasectomy is probably second to cystoscopy (looking in the bladder) as the most frequently performed procedure. Though my practice was specialized in several areas (oncology, endourology, and pediatric urology), I still did more vasectomies during my 31 years of practice than any other procedure (aside from cystoscopy). There was a huge demand among the young healthy couples for vasectomy so among the seven urologists in our network, we each averaged about five a week.

We would schedule them after clinic hours in the evening so that the demand would not affect access to urologic care for other things like cancer, stones, people who can't pee, or people who pee too much and can't control it. We didn't have the time during the day to do proper informed consent, so we did "vasectomy classes" in the evening where a urologist would give an "informed consent" lecture to 25 couples.

I enjoyed doing the group lecture. The men would appear anxious, legs crossed, hands in lap protecting the family jewels, as if I were going to ask one of them to volunteer to demonstrate the technique in front of the audience. Most attended with their wives who sat there reassuring them that "everything is going to be okay," along with something like, "It's nothing compared to giving birth," "It's your turn," or the more stern, "If you think I'm going to get pregnant again, you've got another thing coming!"

Because of the palpable anxiety in the room, I'd start off with a quick joke. "How do you circumcise a whale?"

"Four skin divers!"

Or one that I seemed to enjoy more than the audience, "What's the difference between a hematologist and urologist?"

"One pricks fingers."

Getting a laugh from the audience relaxed them. Once they were relaxed, I'd continue the lecture.

"Part of informed consent has to do with the requirement for sterility after the vasectomy. Urologists have different rules around this issue. Our rule was that after the vasectomy a man must have two neg-ative sperm counts. That means no sperm seen under the microscope after ejaculation. It takes about 20 ejaculations to clear the plumbing of viable sperm. The first negative sperm count is done after two months and the second one after three months. We advise continuing birth control during that three month period. If sperm are still present after the second test, then we advise waiting another month, and en-courage more frequent ejaculation."

It was at this point of the lecture that the look of dread transferred from husband to wife ("Twenty ejaculations in a month! That ain't happening with me, you are on your own pal!") I would try to lighten the mood in the room with another joke, this one dealing with the requirement for sterility after vasectomy.

A man arrives at the 'post-vasectomy clinic' (these places don't ex-ist in reality, but let's assume they do) where he is greeted by a gor-geous nurse. The nurse tells the man "I'm going to help you get your specimen, you'll see, you are going to really enjoy it!"

As they walk down a long hall, the man peaks into several rooms where other men have been supplied with old pornographic material. He's not sure, but it appears that some of them are masturbating.

The gorgeous nurse and man arrive at the end of the hall. She closes the door and asks, "Are you ready?" as she begins to undress.

"Well, uh, I'm not sure," he stammers. "What about all those other guys? How come you aren't giving them this special treatment? Not that I'm refusing, just curious."

'Oh them?' she says. 'They're uninsured."

Vasectomy is usually the first procedure that a first year urology resident learns how to do. For most, even novices, a vasectomy is technically easy. That is, until you realize that you are operating on a man's scrotum, and that he's fully awake and, unless he's had a tranquilizer or shot of whisky, his anxiety is ten plus on a scale of nine. That's what makes it challenging.

The higher the anxiety level, the more difficult the procedure. I'd like to reassure you that after doing over 7,500 vasectomies during my 34 year career, there is absolutely nothing to worry about. There is minimal, if any, pain, complications are extremely rare, and after having one, you will encounter no (as far as I know) unwanted pregnancies.

The Procedure

Recall from Chapter 1 the anatomy of your scrotum. In it are your testicles, which make sperm. The sperm exit the testicles by small tubes at the top back part of the testicles and drain into the epididymis, which is one thin tube squished and coiled into a tube about an inch long. If you uncoiled the tube that makes up the epididymis, it would stretch out to be eight feet long. At the bottom (toward the feet) of the epididymis, the tube becomes the vas deferens. The vas deferens is a firm tube with a diameter of a piece of spaghetti and a small lumen on the inside. The diameter of the lumen is equivalent to a piece of hair.

As each vas leaves the scrotum, the left vas makes a left turn in the groin and the right vas a right turn. They enter the retroperitoneum just inside the right and left pelvic bone, reverse direction, and then head down toward the prostate where they join the right and left seminal vesicles to become the ejaculatory duct. The ejaculatory duct empties into to the prostatic urethra. During ejaculation, the junction of the bladder and prostate (bladder neck) closes and the muscle contractions during orgasm expel the semen. Ninety percent of the semen volume comes from the seminal vesicles, while the remaining ten percent is sperm and prostatic secretions. These secretions from the prostate and seminal vesicles nourish the sperm and enhance fertility. Since a vasectomy interrupts the passage of sperm to the ejaculatory ducts, and since the sperm make up less than five percent of the semen, a vasectomy does not significantly reduce the volume of the ejaculate, which is a common concern among men undergoing vasectomy.

What actually happens when come in for your vasectomy?

A nurse will bring you into an exam room, answer any questions you may have, ask you a few questions about allergies, medications, your medical history, then give you a gown and ask you to get undressed, and put the gown on after s/he leaves the room (you can leave your socks on)

The urologist will come in, ask a few more questions, examine your genitalia, and then scrub your scrotum with an antibacterial soap. It was our practice to have the patients shave their scrotal hair off prior to coming in for vasectomy. The hair gets in the way, so we felt that this was a better option than not shaving. If your urologist asks you to shave, please do not use an electric razor. I'm not joking. I've seen some significant damage to scrotal skin from electric razors. It's okay to use shaving cream, but generally not necessary. If we need to do a touch up of your shave job, we'll do it then. Some urologists may not be bothered by scrotal hair making the shave job up to the doctor doing the procedure.

The urologist feels the vas through the skin, injects a small amount of a local anesthetic in the skin and along each side of the vas. S/he makes a puncture wound, and then uses a skin hook to engage the vas and bring it through the puncture wound. The vas looks like a piece of spaghetti in the shape of an upside down "V." One limb of the "V" is the epididymal end, and the other is the prostate end. There is a small blood vessel (the vasal artery) that runs along the inside of the V, and a sheath of tissue that encases the vas. At this point, more local anesthetic is injected along the limbs of the vas. You can't see the nerve that goes along the course of the vas, but it's there, and injecting additional anesthetic makes the procedure virtually pain free in 99% of cases. The sheath is incised (I usually used a scalpel for this) and the vas is brought through the sheath. The small artery is dissected free of the vas. A small portion (half to 1 cm, or a bit less than a quarter inch to half an inch) of the vas tube is removed. At this point, the cut ends of the vas have to be closed. How this is done is a matter of personal preference. Some urologists use electrocautery by placing a needle electrode down the lumen and allowing the scar to close it off, while others use sutures to tie it off. I've even heard of urologists using titanium surgical clips. Once the ends are occluded, the sheath is used to separate the ends by burying one end in a separate tissue layer using a single dissolvable suture. Ten to 15 minutes after the prep, both sides are done, that's all there is to it. I found that there was no need to suture close the small puncture wound.

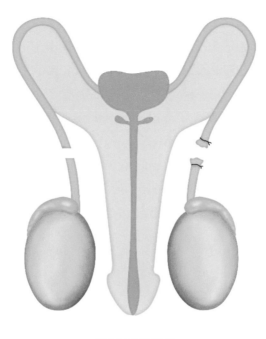

Vasectomy

After the Procedure

After the procedure, a dressing is applied and held in place with tight fitting underwear or a jock strap. The nurse will wheel you out to your car in a wheelchair. **You must not drive home**. In fact, we'd like you not to drive for 24 hours. Once home, we'd like you to stay in bed with an ice pack on top of the dressing continuously for 48 hours. Frozen peas or corn works well for this. I'd recommend having about four packages on hand. When one thaws, put it back in the freezer and apply a fresh one.

Your activities should be limited for a week. That means no sex, running, jumping, working out, yardwork or weightlifting for a week. If you have small children, don't pick them up. Anything that causes increased pressure in the scrotum or within the vas deferens itself can result in swelling, pain, and possible failure of the vasectomy. For pain, all that should be necessary is Tylenol or an NSAID like Advil or Motrin. You can expect some swelling. And, as we've talked about, you are not sterile until you've had two negative sperm counts after 20 ejaculations, both two and three months after the vasectomy. (This requirement for sterility is the one we used in our clinic and may vary from clinic to clinic.) So be sure to continue to use an alternative form of birth control for three months following the procedure, until your urologist has assured you that you're sperm free and sterile.

Vasectomy Failures

The risk of pregnancy after a vasectomy is 1 in 500. Let's talk about that for a minute. If a man has had a vasectomy and has had two negative sperm counts after 20 ejaculations two and three months after the vasectomy, I would say that the risk of that man getting a woman pregnant is virtually nil. I can honestly say that I do not remember a single pregnancy that occurred after a vasectomy that I had done, nor that any of my 18 partners had done if the requirements for sterility were met. If the requirements for sterility were met, and if that man's wife were to become pregnant, a sperm count should be done. Sperm in the ejaculate would be rare. If there are no sperm in that case (and I've never been in that situation), it's probably the case that another man is the father. At that point I'd guess the urologist would have to refer the couple for marriage counseling. If the sperm counts done after vasectomy continue to show sperm, that means one of two things—it means that the two ends of the cut vas have "found each other" and reattached, or it mean that the urologist removed a segment of "something else" and not the vas. When we do vasectomies, the two small segments are sent to the pathologist who looks under the microscope to confirm the fact that two segments of vas were removed. It's possible, I guess, to remove two segments from the same side, leaving the opposite vas intact. I heard of this happening, but I've never seen it. What this does point out is that even though vasectomy is a simple procedure, it may be best to have your vasectomy done by an experienced urologist.

Vasectomy Reversal

Vasectomy is a form of permanent birth control, but vasectomies can be reversed. Six to ten percent men who undergo vasectomy will elect to have it reversed. It may be that the couple changed their minds about having more kids. More often there is a divorce and a second marriage involved. Rarely and unfortunately, a child will die after the father has had a vasectomy, and the couple wants to conceive again.

However, be advised that the reversal procedure—called a vaso-vasostomy—is technically difficult compared to the vasectomy itself, and in the best surgical hands it is only successful 30-70% of the time in producing a pregnancy, depending on how long it has been since the vasectomy. If it's been more than seven years since the vasectomy, the chances of a pregnancy drop to 44%, and after 15 years 30%. And those statistics are generated from a large population of men undergoing reversal (vasovasostomy) done by very experienced and technically excellent urologists

Given how technically difficult a vasectomy reversal procedure is, if you do want a reversal, be sure you find someone who does hundreds of these procedures a year and can tell you what their success rate is. Success is measured two ways—by a return of sperm in the ejaculate and by pregnancy rate. In the best of hands, if the vasectomy was done within the past 10 years, return of sperm in the ejaculate is around 90%, however, the pregnancy rate is more in the range of 70%. The pregnancy rate is better the less time there is between vasectomy and reversal. If there is no sperm in the ejaculate after the vasectomy reversal, then it's not likely that a pregnancy will result. The other factor to consider is that this procedure is expensive and probably not covered by insurance. (The cost of a vasovasostomy at the time of this writing can be anywhere from $5,000 to $15,000.)

Condoms

A few final words about alternatives to vasectomy. The most common form of male birth control is using a condom. But there are few risks of wearing a condom. If the condom is latex, and the man or woman has a latex allergy, there may be an allergic reaction to the condom. The major risk of using a condom for birth control, however, is an unwanted pregnancy. If used "perfectly" and removed after sex "perfectly," the risk of pregnancy is still two percent.[xvi] However, accidents do happen, and condoms are sometimes not put on in time, or sometimes removed too soon, which increases the risk of pregnancy to between five and ten percent.

Male Birth Control Pill

Researchers specializing in contraception have been looking for a male birth control pill for many years. Pharmaceutical male contraceptive research studies have been done on both hormonal and non-hormonal methods. To date, the search for a safe, effective, and well tolerated form of a male birth control pill remains elusive, despite the fact that men are more willing to share the burden of family planning, but still largely unwilling to rely on condoms for contraception. So the burden remains with the female, which is another reason men should consider vasectomy if they are sure they are done fathering children.

Conclusion

Having a vasectomy may be something that you desire, but understandably makes you nervous. I've performed thousands of vasectomies without any problem. I even had one myself. I decided to have a vasectomy because after having our two daughters, my wife developed blood clots—a life-threatening complication—due to birth control pills. One of my partners did my vasectomy on a Friday after we'd finished clinic. I brought a bottle of good scotch, had a little before the procedure, and then he and I shared a little after. Then he drove me home. I had my Labrador Retriever Simon fixed the same day. Simon and I spent the weekend on the couch watching sports. I was back at work Monday morning and took nothing more than a few Advil. It was so simple I wished I had done it 10 years sooner.

In the end, or better yet, the two cut end of the vas deferens, vasectomy offers the safest and most effective form of birth control for both men and women.

CHAPTER 14

Emergencies and Trauma

If you are unlucky enough to have experienced trauma to the genitourinary system, you were likely seen in the emergency room or urgent care. Isolated urologic trauma is rare. Most urologic trauma also involves other organ systems. For example, when there is a significant abdominal injury, ten percent of those injuries involve urologic organs. And fractured lower ribs or a fractured pelvis should put the provider on alert for a possible urologic injury.

Trauma can be categorized as blunt force (such as from motor vehicle accident, a fall, a sports injury like a hard tackle in football, or being hit by a car while walking or riding a bike) or penetrating (gunshot wounds, stabbings, or impalement).

All organs of the GU system are at risk from such injuries, from the top of the kidney to the tip of the penis. Any injury to the lower abdomen or pelvis can injure the bladder, urethra or both. An injury to the lower chest (including fractured ribs) or upper abdomen will usually prompt rapid evaluation in the ER with a CT scan. One sign that ER doctors look for is blood in the urine, either microscopic or blood that can be seen with the naked eye. This may be a sign of an injury to the kidney. Kidney injuries can be mild or severe. Kidney injuries are graded 1 (mild or a contusion, like a kidney bruise) to 4 (severe, which is a shattered kidney or injury to one of the blood vessels going to or from the kidney). Some mild kidney injuries are observed, knowing that they will heal on their own, while other more severe injuries require surgery, which sometimes involves removing the kidney.

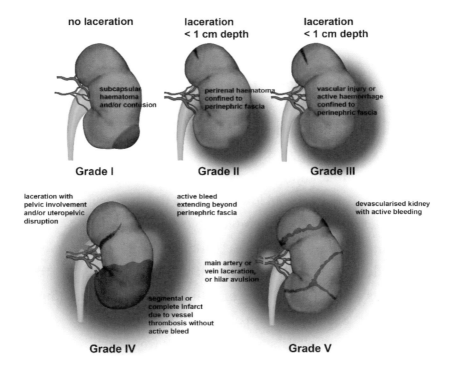

5 grades of blunt renal trauma

Injuries to the lower abdomen and pelvis can result in either a bladder injury, urethral injury, or both. Again, the CT scan is useful in determining if there is an injury to the bladder and/or urethra. Like the kidney, some of these injuries can be observed, while others will require surgery. If the pelvis is fractured in a man, the urethra can be detached or disrupted from the prostate. When this happens, a urologist will need to participate with the orthopedic surgeon to repair the damage. There are many ways to repair this injury dependent on the preferences, experience, and training of the urologist.

But let's consider injuries to the penis, because if you injure that, you want help!

Fracture of the Penis – Talk about Trauma!

You've probably caught on that I spend a lot of time on the golf course, where I encounter no end of questions about my profession, with total strangers divulging their urinary health concerns to me between shots. And there's one topic of conversation that comes up frequently. It goes something like this.

"Can I ask you something Doc?"

"Sure."

"A friend of mine said that he fractured his penis. Is that for real? Does that really happen?"

"Yep, it happens."

"But there aren't any bones in the penis. How can it break?"

"You're right, there are no bones, technically. Boner is kind of a misnomer in fact."

"So how does it break?"

"It's more like a rupture due to excessive force."

"Like really rough sex?"

"Yeah, something like that."

"Do you put a cast on it or what?"

"No, no cast, we do an operation to fix the rupture."

"And what happens after that? Does it stop working?"

"Eventually things usually return to normal. Your shot, we're getting behind." As you can imagine, the opportunity to talk about broken penises tends to distract some players!

A penile fracture can only occur to an erect penis. If you read the chapter on anatomy, you'll recall the penis is basically two long torpedo-shaped sponges (the corpora cavernosa) encased within a tough layer of tissue called the tunica albuginea. When the spongy tissue fills with blood, the penis becomes erect and the tough tunica albuginea stretches.

If there is a sudden and forceful bend in either corporal body, the tunica will rupture, kind of like a blow out on a tire. The penis will immediately become soft, and soon there will be significant swelling as blood flows from the corporal body into the surrounding tissue. The entire penis will turn purple with bruising, a deformity labeled as "an eggplant" deformity. If the urethra is also injured, there may be blood at the urethral opening.

The diagnosis can usually be made just by learning how it happened. A man hears a loud "pop" and his happy erection instantly turned into a most unhappy injury—one obvious by physical exam. When it's uncertain whether the tunica albuginea white fibrous capsule has ruptured or lacerated, an ultrasound or MRI can help make a definitive diagnosis. If this should happen to you, surgery to evacuate the blood that has spilled out into the soft tissue outside of the corporal bodies is generally the best option, and any tears in the tunica albuginea are sutured closed. The repair surgery not only preserves the cosmetic appearance of the penis, but it also maintains sexual function (that would be erections), when compared to conservative (as in no surgery) management.

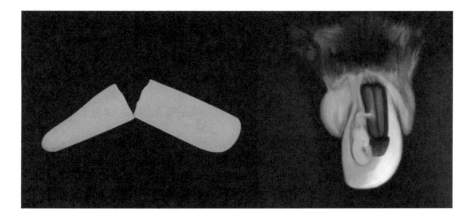

Fractured Penis

note extravasation of blood (white) from traumatic laceration of tunica albuginea of corporal body

Phimosis and Paraphimosis

A discussion about traumatic things that happen to the penis would not be complete without a discussion of phimosis and paraphimosis. Phimosis is when uncircumcised foreskin cannot be retracted behind the glans. Paraphimosis also occurs in uncircumcised men when the foreskin is retracted behind the glans and then gets stuck and cannot be pulled back into its normal position. Phimosis is not an emergency but needs to be attended to, whereas *paraphimosis is an emergency* and should be treated to prevent a worsening situation and pain. Patients suffering from paraphimosis can have considerable swelling and pain and frequently results in a trip to the ER or urologist's office to get the foreskin back to where it belongs.

Phimosis in adult males is a result of scarring and inflammation, and is frequently seen in diabetics, and in men who have had a history of infections of the penis. Moreover, a foreskin that is not retracted can lead to infections (balanitis) and can even cause cancer of the penis later in life. Topical treatment can be tried with steroid cream. If there is another infection present, an anti-fungal can be prescribed as the culprit is usually (but not always), yeast. If all else fails, a circumcision should be done (please see Chapter 2 on circumcision for more information).

Priapism

I coached competitive girls' soccer for 12 years. My friend and co-coach Nick and I were sitting around in a hotel lobby with our team of 13 year old girls waiting to play in a tournament game. There was a TV in the lobby that was on some mindless talk show. At some point a loud commercial came on for Cialis (an erectile dysfunction drug like Viagra or Levitra) that caught the girls' attention. The commercial concluded with, "if your erection lasts longer than four hours, see a doctor" or something like that. One of the girls looked at us and asked, "Four hours! yikes! Does that really happen!?!?). Some of the girls giggled, while others fell silent. I just matter of factly responded, "Not often," and managed to change the subject to soccer and our upcoming game.

A painful and persistent erection of the penis is called priapism, named after the Greek god Priapus who was famous for an enormous, continuous erection. It's nothing you want to have and it is unrelieved by orgasm. If left untreated, tissue damage and even permanent erectile dysfunction (ED) may result. ED drugs, blood thinners, antidepressants (especially trazodone), anti-psychotics, and anti-anxiety drugs, injections into the penis for impotence, as well as illicit drugs (including marijuana, alcohol and cocaine), plus some blood pressure medications can cause priapism.

Thirty-five percent of men with sickle cell anemia are affected by priapism at some time in their life. Other co-morbid medical conditions like a spinal cord injury or injury to the genitals, or leukemia can also cause priapism.

There are two types of priapism—high flow (non-ischemic) and low flow (ischemic). Low flow priapism is painful, high flow usually isn't. To treat priapism, the first step is inserting a needle into the penis to withdraw blood. If the blood is bright right red, it's high flow. If it's purple with clots, it's low flow. High-flow priapism is rare and caused by an injury to the penis. It's may not be as painful as low-flow priapism, but requires emergency treatment nevertheless.

Low-flow priapism can be quite painful. Low-flow priapism can also be caused by injury, but drugs and medications are more common offenders. If you develop a painful erection that won't go away, get to the ER.

Developing an erection that won't go away can be an embarrassing experience and the treatments can be uncomfortable, but you do need treatment. Treatment in the ER usually starts with ice packs applied to the perineum (the space between the scrotum and anus) and penis. Oral medications like pseudoephedrine or terbutaline can be tried while waiting for the on-call urologist to show up. Depending on your medical history and likely cause of the priapism (note that sometimes one can never tell what causes it) your physician will probably try to drain the blood from your penis. This is a procedure called aspiration and involves numbing the penis with a local anesthetic, then injecting a medication (usually phenylephrine) that in most cases of low-flow priapism is effective. When aspiration and phenylephrine fail, the clots and blood can be irrigated out with sterile saline. Sometimes, all those efforts will be unsuccessful in producing flaccid penis, and surgery is necessary. There are a variety of surgical procedures that can be employed to treat priapism that are designed to shunt blood that isn't leaving the penis to tissue or blood vessels that allow the blood to leave thereby producing a flaccid penis.

Successful treatment depends on the duration of the erection. If it's between four and six hours, treatment should be successful. The longer the erection lasts, the riskier it becomes. The goal of treatment is a flaccid penis and normal sexual function in the future.

Catheters

Catheters are necessary and helpful, but they can at times cause problems. Generally speaking, catheters are soft hollow tubes that are used to drain fluid from the body. Catheters are used by a variety of medical specialists, including urologists. In addition to being used to drain fluid (like urine), they can also be placed in spaces to measure certain physiologic metrics (like pressure in a chamber of the heart), or to inject substances for treating certain conditions (like when you want to block blood flow to a part of a certain organ that is bleeding, the interventional radiologist can embolize the blood vessel by placing a coil through a catheter).

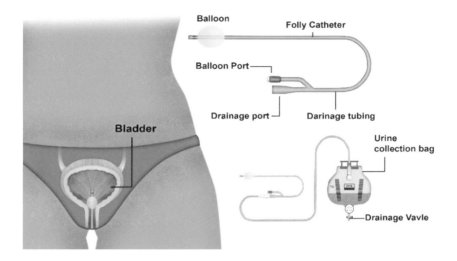

Urinary Foley Catheter

Urinary catheters are like double-edged swords. On the one hand, they are necessary and useful in draining urine from places where urine for whatever reason won't drain. They also provide a way to heal connections (anastomoses) of things that are reconstructed (like the connection between the bladder and urethra after the prostate is removed). On the other hand, (or the other edge of the sword, which I realize may be an uncomfortable metaphor when you are talking about a tube that goes through the penis sometimes), aside from being uncomfortable, when a catheter is displaced or removed before its time, or if it gets obstructed or breaks, it can cause significant problems.

Urologists are experts at urinary catheters. Catheters put into the bladder are called Foley catheters, named after American urologist Frederic Foley, who invented a self-retaining catheter in 1929. Foley developed a catheter with a balloon toward the bladder end of the catheter that could be filled with water through a separate port. It might surprise you to learn that Foley wasn't the first to invent a flexible catheter—Benjamin Franklin invented the first flexible catheter (though without the balloon) in 1752 when he was looking for a way to help his brother James who suffered from bladder and kidney stones. Apparently there wasn't much Ben Franklin didn't succeed at!

Catheters have proven to be remarkable, yet simple, devices for resolving all sorts of issues, and for us urologists, essential to our daily work. Urologists are frequently called about catheter issues Emergency calls come from all sorts of places—emergency rooms, ICUs, med-surg wards, outpatient offices, nursing homes, just about anywhere someone has a catheter, a misadventure can occur.

One of my friends from medical school had his prostate removed for cancer (robotic assisted radical prostatectomy) in Florida. Two days after his surgery, he called me (in Oregon) from the car driven by his wife. He was simultaneously screaming at me and giving directions to his wife to the nearest ER: "You gotta help me......no turn here.....this f..king catheter stopped working and there's.....no damn it, you gotta go on the freeway, can't you drive faster?......blood coming around the catheter!!! My bladder feels like it's going to explode!!!! AGGH, AGGH, AGGH!!!"

Bleeding after a robotic radical prostatectomy is not a common complication, but my buddy had started blood thinners for his heart and he had bled into the bladder. Blood clots in the bladder stopped the urine from draining from the bladder. This is a serious situation because the connection between the bladder and the urethra could leak or come apart. When he finally reached the ER, a urologist was called in, irrigated the clots out, got the catheter working again (it had not been displaced), and the bleeding stopped on its own. Disaster avoided.

Blunt and Penetrating Injuries

Blunt and penetrating injuries can affect any part of the urinary tract from the top of the kidney to the tip of the urethra. Foreign bodies such as a broken off piece of a catheter can also find a home in the urinary tract and cause bleeding, infection, or obstruction. One of the most memorable urinary tract foreign body anecdotes was in 1982 when I was one of three chief residents in urology.

We had just finished Friday evening rounds and were detoxing in the residents' office when the phone rang. "Are you the admitting urologist?" a voice on the other end of the phone asked.

"Who's asking?" I replied.

"I'm Dr So-and-so, Hood River ER. I'm sending a patient to you to be admitted."

"Okay," I answered. "What's the problem?"

"He's got a hardware store up his urethra"

"Whaaat?!?"

"You'll understand when you see the x-ray, I'll send it with him."

"Okay, what's his ETA?"

"He'll be there in a couple of hours"

The patient arrived at 8 pm. Before I went in to meet him and do an H and P (history and physical), I took a look at his x-ray. On the x-ray, in the area of the urethra just under the pubic bone, on the penis side of the prostate, there were four metallic objects. I could make out what looked like an open safety pin, a cotter pin, the spring from a ball point pen, and another unidentifiable metallic object.

"Holy shit!" I said, shocked to see what the referring physician meant by a "hardware store." I'd never seen anything like it, and couldn't imagine the pain the patient was in.

With some trepidation I went into the hospital room and met a seemingly normal man around 40 years of age resting comfortably in bed.

"What brings to the hospital?" I asked him, though I knew full well what had brought him there. I just couldn't imagine how he might characterize this state of his penis.

"I put stuff up my penis and now I can't pee," he casually answered.

"Are you in pain?"

"Not really, but my bladder is pretty full."

"Have you peed blood or pus?"

"No."

"Have you done this before?" I asked him, wondering if a referral for a psyche evaluation was in order.

"Yes, many times, but stuff never gets stuck."

"Mind if I ask why you do it?"

"Cause it feels good, I guess."

To each his own, I figured, as I prepared to examine my friendly but bewildering patient. On physical exam I saw that his bladder was distended. I could feel it way up by his umbilicus (bellybutton), where I saw a scarred white area around his navel.

"What happened here?" I asked.

"Oh that?" he said, with a shrug. "I put gunpowder in there and lit it"

"Yikes, that's like a second or third degree burn. Why?"

"I wanted to see how it felt." He answered my questions as casually as if I were asking about a mild sunburn.

I then asked him my final question before going down to the OR to remove the hardware store, a question I thought quite reasonable considering all that had come before: "Have you ever put anything in your rectum?"

"You mean asshole?" he asked, his tone sounding surprised for the first time.

"Yes," I answered.

He looked me straight in the eye, his eyes widened, and with an angry tone said, "ARE YOU CRAZY!?!?!"

As funny as the story was, it got stranger. We went to the OR. The anesthesiologist did her thing and put him to sleep. I had my back to him checking the instruments on the back table that I would need to attempt removal of the four metallic objects. I was going to try to get them out via the urethra (through the penis) without needing to make an incision, a most challenging feat considering the safety pin was still open. If unsuccessful, I would need to remove the objects from above through the bladder.

With my back turned to the patient, the nurses asked if they could put his legs up in stirrups (that's called low lithotomy position, the same position women have to assume to have a pelvic exam or deliver a baby). After the nurse put his legs up she said, "Hey, look at this doc, he sent you a greeting card." Out of the anus were the bristles of the toothbrush the hospital supplied to patients. I didn't think I was the crazy one.

Fortunately, I was able to remove the objects and spared him an incision. The next day we removed the catheter, and he was able to pee. Before sending him home, I thought that the psychiatrist on call should evaluate him, and possibly admit him, so we called a psychiatry consult. The psychiatrist spent an hour with him and came into the office to report, "He's not psychotic, so I'm not going to transfer him to our service, I think he can go home."

I remember being stunned. Surely he'd do it again. As far as I was concerned, he was a threat to his own safety. So we devised what we thought might solve the issue. We gave him a catheter and told him whenever he got the urge to put something in there, to just use the catheter. We never heard back from him, so I can only hope, he took our advice!

CONCLUSION

I wrote this book in an effort to help patients make better decisions about their urinary healthcare, to have a better sense of their health concerns, and to have informed, shared decision making discussions with their urologists.

When I was actively practicing urology at Kaiser Permanente in Portland, where I had practiced for 31 years, I was bothered by not having enough time to counsel my patients. This was particularly true of men recently diagnosed with new prostate cancer, but it was true for all patients, including those with blood in their urine, kidney stones, people who couldn't pee, or peed too much. All were worried, and all had questions—but there wasn't enough time to answer their questions and concerns in the limited time available.

Men with newly diagnosed prostate cancer deserved better. I had either phoned them with the cancer diagnosis, or they were coming in to get the bad news. Yet I had only 15 minutes for a discussion of the results and what comes next. When done properly, a shared decision making conversation about a new diagnosis of cancer takes at least an hour. That discussion never happened to my or my patient's satisfaction. Instead, they would leave the office confused, depressed, and anxious. Some would go on the internet and Google "treatment of prostate cancer," (as well as "life expectancy," "survival rate" and other dire word strings reflecting their understandable fears). Some would talk to relatives or neighbors who had been through prostate cancer treatment. Whatever they did, they would inevitably return a week or two later full of misinformation, more confusion, and more anxiety.

When I retired in 2014, I needed something to do. I decided to write down all the information I wanted these men (and their families) to know—as well as those who came to me with bladder or renal cancer, infections, urinary problems, or any of a number of things that men commonly suffer but know little about. And I know they want answers because the questions didn't stop with my retirement. To this day I still get a lot of questions, sometimes three or four a week. A lot of these questions are raised on the golf course, often when my mind is far from the topic of urology as I focus on my next shot.

I started playing semi-serious competitive golf. As I've already noted in these chapters, it seemed that every time I got paired with a new guy, after finding out I was a urologist, questions inevitably followed. "Hey doc, my last PSA was 5, should I be worried?" Or "I've had lots of stones, lots of surgery and procedures for my stones, is there anything I can do to stop them?" Or "I had bladder cancer and they took my bladder out a couple of years ago. Did I really have to go through all that?" or "I peed blood last week and I couldn't get into to see a urologist for another six weeks, should I get in sooner?" And there were guys who I never met who would say, "I just got my prostate biopsy back and I have cancer. Can I buy you lunch so we can talk about what to do?"

In 2015 I started volunteering for the M.A.V.E.N. project (Medical Advice Volunteer Expert Network https://www.mavenproject.org/)as

a clinical consultant. The MAVEN project provides health consultation to over 200 clinics for the uninsured in 19 states. None of these clinics have specialists, they are all staffed by primary care providers (generalists, internists, family practitioners, nurse practitioners, and physician assistants). Whenever these PCPs require specialty consultation for their patients, they submit an electronic consult. Almost every specialty you can imagine is represented by a volunteer physician in that specialty. As I started responding to these requests for help with urology, I realized that it wasn't just the guys on the golf course who had questions—the PCPs were thirsting for information and guidance.

So, I flipped open my laptop and started writing about the common urologic conditions that brought men to my office, the stuff I was asked about both on the golf course and by the MAVEN PCPs. When I was done, if someone on the golf course asked me a question, I'd send them the relevant chapter. When a MAVEN PCP working in a free clinic wanted a consult on a kidney tumor, I'd send the chapter on kidney tumors. Soon, the feedback I received made it clear that I needed a better way to disseminate this information to those who had questions. And that brings me to you.

This book is for you. I'm assuming you are a nonmedical person with a urologic problem, or someone you care about has a urologic issue. You may be one of the guys I play golf with who I noticed peeing every other hole and then says to me, "my urologist wants to do some new procedure on my prostate to help me pee better, have you heard of it? Did you do that when you were in practice?" You maybe you've seen blood in your urine, or you may be thinking about getting a vasectomy, just in case. Or you may have been told there's a mass in your kidney, a tumor in your bladder, or your biopsy shows prostate cancer. Whatever your issue, I know you're concerned, and I know you want—and need—more information.

Whatever inspired you to open this book, however, it is not meant to substitute for a conversation between you and your doctor. I've written these chapters to supplement the conversation most doctors do not have half the time to provide you – time you need, and time that our modern healthcare system has made nearly impossible for them to provide. The material I've gone over in this book is meant to help you wade through the millions of "hits" you will get when you Google your problem whether, "should I get a PSA?" or "what does it mean if there's blood in my urine?" If anything, *this book will save you and your doctor time.*

I have also tried to be frank without alarming you, as well as evidence based. Personal bias enters into every doctor's decision – one might favor one way of taking care of a problem over another, or one might think that one drug is superior to another, or that one way of taking a kidney stone out is superior to an alternative. This physician bias comes into play frequently. Sometimes treatments are equal, but the risks are different. Sometimes one treatment will be better than an alternative but has different and potentially more dangerous risks. And your values, needs, and preferences are different from the next patient's. I've tried taking all these factors into consideration, and I've tried letting you know when I am being biased (early detection of prostate cancer using PSA, for example), where that bias comes from, and why I think it's important.

Decisions you make about your urologic health are not easy. There's a lot to know, and a lot to consider. Most times decisions are best when patients fully understand their issue, what the possible options are for addressing the problem, and the potential risks and benefits of the potential treatments. My hope is that this book will help you and your doctor share in making the best decision for you and for the people you love.

APPENDIX

Prostate anatomy video:

vimeo.com/user68317809/
password: prostate18

Late breaking news:

PSA chapter Man's Guide: Proclarix for clinically significant prostate cancer
https://bjui-journals.onlineli-
brary.wiley.com/doi/abs/10.1111/bju.15998
combined with MRI, improved specificity and sensitivity.

BPH chapter Man's Guide re Rezum a relatively new non-invasive method of treating benign prostate enlargement: https://onlineli-brary.wiley.com/doi/abs/10.1002/pros.24508. Aquablation is another new technique for benign enlargement of the prostate and is best discussed here
https://pubmed.ncbi.nlm.nih.gov/35150215/

Bladder Cancer Chapter both Guides: This is a good article on current management of muscle invasive bladder cancer (MIBC).

Renal Masses: This is a great summary article about current treatment of the most common kidney cancer, renal cell carcinoma or hypernephroma. https://www.cancer.gov/types/kidney/hp/kidney-treatment-pdq. There have been significant changes in treating advanced RCCa with the addition of valuable new chemo and immune agents. Many of these new promising agents are undergoing clinical trials. If you have advanced RCCa, I would advise seeing an oncologist who can discuss these clinical trials with you.

GLOSSARY

active surveillance (AS) – after diagnosing low risk prostate cancer, AS is a protocol for monitoring the cancer using PSA, MRI, and possible repeat biopsies. A third of patients on AS will progress to higher risk, potentially dangerous cancers, at which point definitive treatment should be considered.

adenocarcinoma - malignant cancer that originates from glandular tissue

adjuvant, neo-adjuvant chemotherapy - additional therapy added to another cancer treatment, for example, radiation after surgery. Neo-adjuvant therapy is additional therapy that is given before another therapy, for example, chemotherapy before surgery.

adrenal glands - triangular shaped glands about 1" high and 3" long composed of an inner (medulla) and outer (cortex) layer. The medulla makes adrenaline and noradrenaline, while the cortex makes other hormones that control blood pressure, part of the immune system, and other metabolic processes. You normally have two, one on top of each kidney.

adrenaline (noradrenaline) - stress hormones (same as epinephrine and norepinephrine) produced by adrenal glands. These hormones are secreted during stress ("flight or fight" response), and play a role in heart rate, breathing rate, sugar and carbohydrate metabolism, and muscle function.

adult polycystic kidney disease (APKD) - An inherited genetic (autosomal dominant) disease affecting 1 in 1000 people characterized by multiple cysts in both kidneys. Symptoms usually show up in people in their 30s and 40s.

alpha blocker - typically these are drugs that lower blood pressure. Tamsulosin (Flomax) is a specific type of alpha blocker that does not lower blood pressure primarily, but rather relaxes smooth muscle of urinary tract organs (ureters, bladder neck, prostate). The main use of alpha blockers in urology is to aid in urination, bladder emptying, and relaxing the ureter to aid in stone passage.

anastomosis - attachment between two structures, such as bladder to urethra, ureter to ureter, blood vessels, renal pelvis to ureter, segments of intestine to intestine, ureter to intestine, and more.

anatrophic nephrolithotomy - an open procedure through a flank incision for very large kidney stones in which the solid tissue of the kidney is bivalved to get the stone out. This procedure has been rarely done since 1985

angiomyolipoma of the kidney- a solid benign mass of the kidney made up of fat, blood vessels and muscle. Diagnosis is often made by

CT scan that shows fat in the mass. AMLs can grow and although benign, if > 5.0 can cause life threatening bleeding. Usually asymptomatic, but when large can be painful.

appendix epididymis - a tiny (match head) developmental remnant attached to the epididymis that you can't feel and generally does not cause problems. However, if it twists it will hurt. The pain is controlled with non-steroidal anti-inflammatory medication (such as Motrin or Advil) and usually resolves in a few days.

appendix testes - same as appendix epididymis but attached to the testes between the top of the testes and epididymis.

aquablation - a new procedure recently approved for treatment of bladder outlet obstruction due to prostate enlargement using a high pressure waterjet that destroys prostate tissue while monitoring the waterjet with an ultrasound in the rectum. A robotic arm precisely aids in the delivery of the waterjet.

arteriole - a small arterial blood vessel branch off an artery before draining into a capillary.

artery - a blood vessel that carries blood and oxygen from the heart to tissues and organs in the body.

asymptomatic - without symptoms.

atrophy – when an organ or tissue wastes away or shrinks as a result of being deprived of oxygen, blood, and nutrients.

B-sitosterol - a chemical that is found in plants (avocados, nuts), vegetable oil, and salad dressing. It is also found in some over the counter preparations designed to help men urinate by reducing prostate swelling.

bacteria - single cell organisms seen only under the microscope, lacking a nucleus, and present in the large intestine where they do more good than harm. There are many different types and shapes and present in many environments including water, soil, and organic matter.

balanitis - infection or inflammation of the head of the penis more common in uncircumcised men (particularly diabetics) that presents as pain, swelling, redness, and occasionally purulent discharge.

benign - not cancer, not harmful.

BOO - bladder outlet obstruction. The bladder outlet is where the bladder is attached to the prostate.

BPH - a pathologic term that stands for benign prostatic hyperplasia. BPH produces an overgrowth of prostate tissue that results in squeezing the passageway of urine though the prostate.

BUN - blood urea nitrogen. Protein is broken down in the liver. Urea is a waste product of this process. The kidneys filter the blood and add urea and nitrogen to urine. Urea nitrogen levels rise in the blood when the kidneys aren't working properly and in cases of dehydration, heart failure, high protein diet, and certain medication.

bacteriuria - bacteria in the urine, sometimes associated with infection and inflammation, other times without infection.

bilirubin - a blood test that measures a byproduct of hemoglobin break down in the liver.

CBC - a blood test that stands for complete blood count that measures the number of red blood cells, white bloods cells, and platelets.

calcium oxalate - crystals that are made from a salt of calcium and oxalate and form the most common urinary tract stone.

calculus - a stone formed from mineral salts and organic material found in the kidney, ureter, bladder, prostate, urethra (can also form in the gall bladder, pancreas, ducts draining both liver and pancreas).

cancer - a malignant growth or tumor that results from uncontrolled growth of abnormal cells, glands, and tissue.

carcinoma in situ (CIS) - growth of cancer cells in the tissue layer of origin seen under the microscope. For our purposes, the lining of the bladder, ureters, prostatic urethra, or hollow lining of the kidney collecting system. Can be seen in other organ systems in which the term takes on different meaning (breast, lung, skin, for example).

castrate level testosterone - testosterone after castration, usually less than 50 ng/dL. This low level of testosterone reflects testosterone made by the adrenal glands. Androgen ablation therapy for prostate cancer with Lupron for example, has a goal of testosterone < 50ng/dL

checkpoint inhibitor chemotherapy - your immune system normally has "checkpoints" that prevent an over response to normal tissues and organs in your body. The checkpoints also prevent your immune system from responding to cancer and tumors. These are drugs that block or inhibit the "checkpoints" and allow your immune system to eradicate the tumor or cancer cells. These drugs have been effective in treating cancers like melanoma and some lung cancers. Over the past

10 years ongoing clinical trials are looking at treating a variety of urological cancers, particularly renal cell carcinoma and bladder cancer.

clinically significant prostate cancer - a lesion that is intermediate to high risk based on Gleason score of 7-10 with a volume > 0.5 cm3, or documented spread outside the prostate.

chemo/chemotherapy - a variety of drugs that all have different mechanisms of action designed to treat cancer. The main type of chemo is "cytotoxic," which means "kills cells."

citrate - a salt of citric acid which inhibits calcium stone formation. An antioxidant, citrate is found in a variety of fruits and vegetable (lemons, grapefruit, avocado, prunes, and more).

corpora cavernosa - the two erectile compartments that comprise most of the penis. Inside is spongy tissue that fills with blood during an erection. Both corporal bodies are covered by a tough outer layer called the tunica albuginea.

creatinine - a chemical that can be measured in blood and urine. Creatinine is a byproduct of the chemical process of energy production by muscles. Healthy kidneys filter blood and add creatinine to urine, which is excreted (peed out) as a waste product. When kidneys are not working properly or in the case of severe dehydration, creatinine levels to rise in the blood.

cryoablation - a process of freezing tissue or tumors to super cold temperatures that results in cellular death. Used in urology for treatment of prostate and kidney tumors.

CT scan - computerized tomography commonly called a "cat scan." Uses images of multiple x-rays taken in a variety of directions, then fed into a computer that reconstructs the image to resemble a facsimile of tissue, organs, and bones of your body.

CT urogram - computerized tomography (CT) to evaluate the urinary tract consisting of kidneys, ureters, bladder, and prostate (men). During the urogram phase of the study, x-ray dye or contrast is injected in a vein in the arm or hand and is then taken up by the kidneys (or kidney tumor) and excreted into the urinary tract.

cyst - a fluid contained by a smooth, thin walled sac-like structure.

cystectomy, simple - removal of the urinary bladder (simple).

cystectomy, radical - removal of the urinary bladder and prostate in a man; removal of the urinary bladder and roof of the vagina, urethra, and the uterus in a female.

cystinuria - cystine is an amino acid similar to lysine, ornithine, arginine. Cystinuria is an inherited disorder in which large amount of cystine and cystine crystals are in the urine and form stones.

cystoscopy - a procedure done with a flexible fiberoptic scope to enable the urologist to look at the inside of the urethra, bladder, and prostate.

cystitis - infection or inflammation (or both) of the bladder.

cystometrogram - a procedure done with a catheter in the bladder that measures pressure in the bladder as the bladder fills with saline.

double J stent (JJ stent) - a thin flexible plastic hollow tube that resides in the ureter with one "J" or curl in the hollow part of the kidney, and the other J in the bladder. The stent allows drainage of urine from kidney to bladder in order to bypass obstruction from stones, tumor, or scar tissue.

dihydrotestosterone (DHT) - a male hormone that is a byproduct of testosterone metabolism. Testosterone is converted to dihydrotesterone by an enzyme called 5 alpha reductase. This conversion is blocked by drugs called 5 alpha reductase inhibitors (Proscar/finasteride, Avodart/dutersteride).

diverticulum - a sac or a tube that forms because of a weakness in the wall of a hollow organ or occurs because of increased pressure in that organ. Can also be congenital. Diverticulum can be found in the kidney, ureter, or bladder, and can vary in size from tiny (1/4 inch) to large (tennis ball).

ductuli efferentes - small thin tubes that conduct sperm from the testicle to head of epididymis located at the top back part of the testicle.

ejaculatory duct - the small tube that drains into the internal portion of the prostate (prostatic urethra) after the vas deferens and seminal vesicle join to form it.

embolization – a procedure to stop the flow of blood using tiny coils, beads, or sponges to therapeutically stop the flow of blood to an organ.

endoscope - a fiber optic instrument that is used to examine the inside of a body cavity.

endourology - the specialized area of urology that employs minimally invasive techniques using endoscopes to treat a variety of problems, particularly urinary tract stones.

epididymis - a structure the size of a caterpillar attached to the top back part of the testicle. Within the structure is a tightly coiled tube. Sperm mature and are temporarily stored within the epididymis.

epididymitis - infection or inflammation (or both) of the epididymis

ESWL - extracorporeal (outside the body) shockwave lithotripsy (break up stones), a non-invasive procedure that uses shockwaves focused using x-rays or ultrasound to break up stones in the urinary tract (has also been used in the biliary tract draining the liver, and the pancreas).

erythropoietin - a hormone made in the kidney that stimulates production of red blood cells in bone marrow.

external sphincter - the skeletal muscle of the pelvic floor through which the urethra passes. You open and close the external sphincter if you stop and start your urinary stream. You can strengthen the external sphincter doing Kegel's exercises. The external sphincter is the remaining sphincter that maintains continence after the prostate is removed.

5 alpha reductase inhibitor - drugs that prevent the conversion of testosterone to dihydrotestosterone like Proscar (finasteride) and Avodart (dutesteride).

fluoroscopy - a continuous x-ray beam like an x-ray "video."

fungus - a microorganism more complicated than bacteria or viruses. Certain fungi are pathogenic, meaning they can cause disease. examples are candida (yeast), and coccidioimycosis (Valley Fever).

GI - gastrointestinal. The GI tract includes the esophagus, stomach, small intestine, large intestine, rectum, liver, biliary system, and pancreas.

glans penis - the head of the penis. the female equivalent is the clitoris.

Gleason grade – A method of evaluating prostate cancer using a scale from one to five, measuring the microscopic appearance of the cells and how the cells are arranged.

Gleason score - the most common appearing grade plus the second most common appearing grade. The scoring system corresponds to how aggressive a particular prostate cancer is, and the speed at which that cancer grows and spreads. A Gleason score of 6 is low risk, 7 intermediate, and 8-10 high risk.

glucose - a simple sugar made of 6 carbon atoms that is an important energy source for many organisms.

hematuria, microscopic - blood in urine that can be seen only under the microscope.

hematuria, gross - blood in urine that can be seen with the naked eye and ranging from light pink to dark red with blood clots

hemorrhagic cyst - a cyst in the kidney that has blood in it. A hemorrhagic cyst has characteristic ultrasound, CT, and MRI appearance.

HIFU - High Intensity Focused Ultrasound that is used to treat prostate cancer. Is not recommended for firstline treatment of prostate cancer, but rather as an alternative to active surveillance, or in cases in which first line therapy has failed. The treatment is done through the rectal wall using an ultrasound probe the heats the cancer to 190º F or 90º C.

hydrocele - a fluid (serum) filled sac in the scrotum that contains the testicle and epididymis. In an infant, a hydrocele is always associated with a hernia.

ileus - small or large bowel paralysis in response to abdominal or retroperitoneal pain, toxins, or surgery.

ileal conduit/ileal loop - a segment of small intestine (usually ilium) to which are attached the ureters draining urine from the kidneys. One end is closed, and the other end fixed to the skin, which is called a stoma of ileostomy.

infection - a state in which a bug (usually bacteria or virus) causes illness in a host.

inflammation - your body's immune response to infection or injury, can be chronic or acute.

internal sphincter - one of three valves in men that are responsible for continence (the prostate and external sphincter are the other two) and in women it's one of two valves (the external sphincter being the 2nd). It is located at the junction of the bladder and prostate in men, and bladder and urethra in women. It is an involuntary sphincter made of smooth (as opposed to skeletal) muscle.

intra-corporal injection therapy - a treatment for ED wherein medication is injected directly into the spongy tissue of the penis. Corporal refers to the corpora cavernosa of the penis.

intra-vesical therapy - Drugs (chemotherapy, immunotherapy, other) that are instilled into the bladder, typically for treating bladder cancer and interstitial cystitis.

IVP/IU - Intravenous pyelogram/intravenous urogram, a procedure more of historical interest because it's been replaced by CTU, rarely done anymore, wherein dye is injected into a vein followed by x-tomography of the kidneys, then sequential x-rays of the bladder.

ketones - a breakdown product of fat metabolism. When you are fasting and your body has exhausted its supply of carbohydrates (sugars, glucose, etc.) for energy, the liver will breakdown fat for energy. The by products are ketones, which causes them to show up in the urine. Small amounts of ketones on urine analysis are normal.

leukocyte - A white blood cell made by bone marrow important in fighting infection and other ailments. Part of the immune and inflammatory response to a variety of problems.

laparoscope - a thin instrument with a camera and a light on the end. The camera displays an image on a video monitor (TV screen). A "working channel" is part of the scope and allows surgeons to pass instruments that allow surgeons to perform a variety of tasks.

laparoscopic surgery - a form of "minimally invasive" (MIP) abdominal and/or retroperitoneal surgery done using laparoscopes through one-inch incisions.

lithotripsy - any procedure that results in "breaking up stones."

lumen - a tube, tubular organ, channel, or cavity.

LUTS - lower urinary tract symptoms, such as frequent urination, having the urge to void, pain with urination, slow trickling urinary stream, feeling of incomplete emptying, and getting up at night to pee.

malignant - refers to cancer, meaning the cells grow in an uncontrolled way. The cells have a typical appearance under the microscope. Tumors made up of malignant cells are more prone to grow rapidly and spread to other parts of the body.

margin positive disease - after a tumor specimen is removed the outer edges are marked with a special ink. The pathologist then examines tissue from the specimen in a systematic way. If the cancer cells abut the inked margin then there is margin positive disease.

metastatic - cancer that has spread via blood or lymph to other parts or organs of the body. For many urologic cancers, that means lymph nodes and bones, but does not exclude other organs (liver, lung, brain, other).

metastatic workup - a series of tests that are done to see if cancer has spread, typically to include a bone scan, CT scans or MRI scans of chest and abdomen (and sometimes head), PET scans, and PSMA scans.

MIBC - muscle invasive bladder cancer. Bladder cancer (usually transitional cell cancer) that invades muscle.

minimally invasive procedure (MIP) - surgery or other procedures done with limited amount of cutting, or through very small incisions.

Examples include robotic laparoscopic surgery, cryotherapy, and several outpatient procedures for BPH. Hopeful benefits are less pain, fewer complications, quicker recovery time, less scarring, less stress on the immune system, smaller or no incision (ESWL).

mucosa - the lining layer of any hollow organ. Urinary bladder, ureter, kidney, stomach, intestine (large and small), all have a mucosal lining layer. The glands of this lining layer make mucous.

neoadjuvant therapy - for cancer, therapy done before the main therapy, such as chemotherapy done before surgery, in order to shrink the tumor or make it more susceptible to treatment (e.g., hormone ablative neoadjuvant therapy before radiation for prostate cancer).

neobladder - a "new" or replacement urinary bladder constructed out of intestine. A form of urinary diversion. When the pouch (neobladder) is attached to the urethra, near normal urination may resume. This is called "orthotopic." When the pouch is attached to the abdominal skin and a bag to collect urine is not necessary, it's called a "continent neobladder."

nephron - one of the millions of microscopic units of the kidney that filters blood, removes wastes, regulates electrolytes and other bodily chemicals, and then adds to what is not needed water to make urine.

nephrostomy tube - or "neph tube" is a soft flexible tube ranging in size from 1/4" to 1/2" (in adults) that directly drains urine from the internal hollow part of the kidney through a small incision, usually in the back.

neurotransmitter - a chemical made by nerve cells that sends a message to other nerve cells, muscle cells, and organs. The specific message results in a specific effect. For example, a neurotransmitter is sent via nerves to the penis that results in an erection.

NMIBC - non-muscle invasive bladder cancer (see MIBC).

nocturia - urination during the night.

nocturnal penile tumescence - spontaneous erections that occur during the night. The word tumescence means "swollen."

NSAID - non-steroidal anti-inflammatory, examples are ibuprofen, Advil, Motrin, aspirin.

OAB - overactive bladder.

oncologist - a doctor (MD or DO) who specializes in the diagnosis and treatment of cancer.

orthotropic neobladder - an internal reservoir for urine that replaces the urinary bladder. It is normally constructed from small intestine. Orthotropic means that it is attached to the urethra so that the patient urinates in the usual way.

osteoporosis - weak, fragile, brittle bones that results from loss of bone tissue, caused by hormone changes like androgen deprivation therapy, vitamin D and/or calcium deficiency.

oxalate - a salt of oxalic acid the occurs in a variety of plants, vegetables, nuts, and other edible food. In urine when combined with calcium forms calcium oxalate stones.

paraphimosis – a condition in uncircumcised males when the foreskin is trapped behind the head of the penis. When prolonged and the foreskin has not reduced to the normal position, there can be significant pain, swelling, and even injury to the tissue of the penis.

partial nephrectomy - a surgery in which a part of the kidney that contains a tumor or disease is removed.

PDE5 inhibitors - phosphodiesterase inhibitor. A class of drugs used to treat ED (Viagra, Levitra, and Cialis) by blocking an enzyme in the walls of blood vessels causing blood vessels to dilate, which increases the flow of blood to certain areas of the body, including the penis.

percutaneous nephrostolithotmy (PERC or PNL) - a surgical procedure done through a small incision in the back in which a tube is passed into the kidney to remove stones. Usually reserved for larger stones, obstructions downstream from the kidney, or when other less invasive methods are not likely to succeed.

perineum - the area of the body between the scrotum and anus in men, and the vagina and anus in women.

peritoneal cavity - the cavity in the abdomen that contains the stomach, liver, small intestines, spleen, etc. contained by a membrane called the peritoneum.

Peyronie's Disease - a non-cancerous condition the affects the penis due to a dense and sometimes painful scar that occurs on the covering tissue (tunica aluginea) of the spongy erectile tissue of the penis (corpora spongiosum). The scar can cause a significant curve or bend in the penis and make intercourse difficult.

pH - the acid base status of fluids in the body - blood, urine, intestinal contents, measured on a scale of 1 (very acid) to 14 (very base), where a pH of 7 is neutral. Normal pH for blood is 7.4. Normal urine pH ranges from 4.5 to 8.

phimosis - a condition in uncircumcised males older than 5 years old in which the foreskin is tight or stuck and cannot be retracted.

placebo - a pill, treatment, or procedure that has no physiologic effect, such as a sugar pill or water, or a fake operation. Used as a "control" when evaluating new drugs or procedures.

posterior repair - a procedure done on the floor of the vagina to fix prolapse of the rectum frequently done in conjunction with a mid-urethral sling.

post vas pain syndrome - persistent scrotal pain three months after vasectomy possibly caused by back pressure, sperm leak, nerve compression, or inflammation.

post void residual (PVR) - the amount of urine in the bladder after urination measured by ultrasound or catheterization.

PCP - primary care provider (Family Practice MD, Internist, Physician Assistant, Nurse Practitioner, Pediatrician).

premature ejaculation - generally speaking, ejaculation that occurs sooner than either participant likes. International guidelines define it as regular and frequent ejaculation that occurs within one minute of entering a partner.

premature detumescence - loss of erection prior to orgasm and ejaculation that may be a sign of impaired circulation.

priapism - a medical emergency defined as a prolonged and often-times painful erection that does not go down after orgasm and ejaculation.

psychogenic impotence - Inability to obtain or maintain an erection when all vascular, neurologic, hormonal parameters, and nocturnal penile tumescent testing is normal.

PSMA scan - A special type of PET scan (positive emission tomography) that looks for spread of prostate cancer. A special tracer chemical is injected 60 minutes prior to the PET scan. The tracer binds to prostate cancer cells and shows up as bright spots on imaging. A CT is done at the same time to localize the cancer.

PSA - Prostate specific antigen. A protein made by benign and cancerous prostate cells. Can be measured in blood and/or tissue. Exists in serum bound to other protein and unbound or "free" PSA.

pyelonephritis - inflammation of the kidney usually from a bacterial infection that presents as flank pain, and usually fever, and sweats, and sometimes nausea and vomiting.

pyelolithotomy - an operation in which a stone is removed from the renal pelvis, the hollow internal part of the kidney that stores and then transports urine from the kidney to the ureter.

radiation oncologist - an MD or DO who specializes in treating cancers using radiation therapy.

radiation therapy - treatment of disease, particularly cancer, using x-rays and a variety of other forms of radiation.

re-canalization - when a bodily tube or channel like the vas deferens is blocked or obstructed and a new channel is created to restore flow in the tube.

renal cell carcinoma (RCC, same as adenocarcinoma of the kidney, and clear cell carcinoma) - most common type of kidney cancer that is the result of uncontrolled glandular tissue of the kidney producing a solid tumor.

renal colic - severe flank pain which is the is the result of blockage along the course of the ureter from where it joins the kidney down to the bladder. Causes of obstruction include stones, scars, congenital narrowing of the ureter (UPJ or UVJ obstruction), or pathology that compresses the ureter from outside the ureter (enlarged lymph nodes for example).

renal pelvis - the central hollow area of the kidney where urine collects before it is transported to the ureter.

renin - an enzyme made and stored in the kidney that is important in blood pressure control.

Rezum - A minimally invasive procedure for treatment of prostate enlargement that uses hot steam to denature prostate tissue. This results in shrinkage of the prostate and a larger passageway for urine.

retrograde ejaculation - ejaculate that goes backwards into the bladder from the prostate rather than out through the urethra. A common side effect of a class of drugs called alpha blockers (tamsulosin/Flomax for example).

retrograde pyelogram - an x-ray study in which radiopaque contrast is injected into the ureter from the bladder into the kidney collecting system. Usually done as in conjunction with cystoscopy.

retroperitoneum - the space behind the abdominal cavity (peritoneum) that contains large arteries and veins (aorta and vena cava), lymph nodes, kidneys, adrenal glands, pancreas.

robotic surgery - In urology, surgery done by attaching laparoscopic instruments and a camera to multiple robotic arms that are controlled by a surgeon sitting at a console.

saturation biopsies of the prostate - 10-14 tissue samples are obtained during a standard prostate biopsy procedure under local anesthesia. When circumstances dictate the need for more tissue to diagnose a suspected prostate cancer, as many as 50 biopsies are done, usually under general anesthesia.

saw palmetto - a natural supplement used to treat lower urinary tract symptoms cause by prostate enlargement. It comes from the fruit of the Serenoa repens tree.

seminal vesicle - a pair of glands that empty into the prostate via the ejaculatory ducts after joining with each vas deferens. 95% of the ejaculate comes from the semen made in the seminal vesicles.

sepsis - a consequence of a life threatening infection in which the body's immune system response damages tissue and organs.

septic shock - a result of severe sepsis in which there is loss of blood pressure.

serosa - the outer membrane that covers organs of the body like the urinary bladder.

shared decision making - an exchange between patients and doctors working together to make decisions regarding tests, treatments, and care plans. The discussions involve weighing risks and benefits of treatments based on evidence and possible outcomes. Patient values, lifestyles, and expectations are taken into account.

seminiferous tubules - microscopic tubules within the testes that serve as a conduit for sperm. The cells that make up the tubules produce sperm.

skeletal muscle - also known as striated muscle, attached to the bony skeleton and contracts in response to volitional nerve stimulation.

smooth muscle - muscle that occurs in internal organs not under voluntary control.

spermatocoele - a benign fluid filled cyst between the top back part of the testes and head of the epididymis that contains a milky white fluid and possibly sperm.

squamous cell carcinoma - squamous cells make up the outer layer of skin, so cancer that originates from these cells is usually a skin cancer, however, squamous cell carcinoma can rarely be seen in the urinary bladder. It is the most common type of cancer of the penis involving the glans and or foreskin.

staghorn calculus - a large branched kidney stone that is often associated with an infection. A struvite stone can be a staghorn calculus and is made up of ammonium, phosphate, and magnesium. Also known as 'triple phosphate' stone.

steroid - organic compounds that include certain manufactured drugs, natural occurring hormones, and vitamins.

stoma, catheterizable stoma - a hollow organ like a segment of intestine that is usually attached to the skin. If one needs to place a catheter through the stoma to empty the contents of whatever needs to be transferred out of the body, it's called a catherizable stoma.

stomal therapist - a nurse who is an expert at taking care of stomas, the skin surrounding the stoma, and the appliances (drainage bags) that are sometimes necessary to collect bodily contents.

testicular torsion - when the testes rotate around (1-3 times) within the scrotum twisting the cord and occluding the blood supply to the testes.

testosterone - male steroid hormone responsible for libido, sexual function, and male sexual characteristics.

transitional cells - type of cells that line the urinary bladder, ureter, and hollow collecting unit of the kidney (renal pelvis and calyces).

transitional cell cancer - also known as urothelial cell cancer, most common type of cancer of the bladder, ureter, internal portion of the kidney.

TriMix - a mixture of three drugs that are injected into the spongy tissue of the penis to treat erectile disfunction. The three drugs are papavarine, phentolamine, and alprostadil.

tumor - an abnormal mass or swelling of body tissue that can be benign or malignant.

tumor markers in urine (NMP-22, FISH) - proteins produced by cancer cells that can be measured in urine or blood. NMP stands for nuclear matrix protein, and FISH stands for fluorescence in situ hybridisation, and is a measure of genetic changes in DNA of tumors. Both of these tests are used to detect bladder cancer.

tunica albuginea - the dense tissue that encapsulates each spongy body (corpora cavernousa) of the penis (see Peyronie's Disease).

TURBT - transurethral (through the urethra) resection of a bladder tumor. An endoscopic procedure done through the urethra wherein a bladder tumor is removed. Any bleeding can be stopped using electrocautery through the same instrument.

TURIP - transurethral incision of the prostate. Endoscopic incisions are made at 5 and/or 7 o'clock at the bladder neck junction of the bladder and prostate to enlarge the passageway and let urine pass more freely.

TURP - transurethral (through the urethra) resection of the prostate. A surgical procedure done through the penile urethra that removes "the pulp of the orange" by systematically resecting the tissue in small segments. The segments are irrigated out of the bladder.

TVO procedure - a type of urethral sling procedure that places tension free urethral tape at slightly different exit incisions.

TVT procedure/tension-free vaginal tape - a procedure designed to provide support for the urethra so that when a cough or laugh or other increase of abdominal pressure occurs, the sphincters are in a position to work properly, and no leak occurs.

ultrasound - a painless imaging technique that that uses sound waves and involves no contrast and no x-rays. The sound waves create a picture called a sonogram of structures and organs in the body.

UPJ - ureteropelvic junction. Where the hollow internal part of the kidney called the renal pelvis joins the first part of the ureter (closest to the head).

UVJ - ureterovesical junction. Where the end of the ureter joins and empties into the bladder.

ureter - the straw-like hollow tube measuring about a foot in length that drains urine from the kidney into the bladder.

ureteral orifice - the end of the ureter as it ends in the bladder. On the floor of the bladder is a triangular shaped structure called the trigone. Each ureteral orifice is seen as a tiny hole and is the entrance to the ureter located at 2 of the 3 corners of the triangle.

ureteroscope - a fiber optic instrument with a camera on the end to allow an image to be displayed on a TV monitor. Usually flexible (but occasionally rigid), it has two working channels, one for saline, and the other for instruments like stone baskets or forceps.

ureteroscopic lithotripsy - a procedure that breaks up stones under direct vision using ureteroscope.

urethra - the tube through which the bladder drains urine.

urethral meatus - The hole at the end of the urethra - on the end of the penis in males, and top part of the vagina in females.

urethral stricture - a narrowing or scar within the urethra. A stricture can be very short (1-2 mm) or very long (> 2-3 cm).

uric acid - a breakdown product of purines responsible for stones of the same name and gout. Purines are found in a variety of foods (beans, peas, beer, liver, anchovies) and is a normal metabolite in the body.

urine cytology - a way of detecting cancer from the lining of the kidney, ureter, or bladder in which the cells are prepared in a special way and examined by the pathologist under the microscope.

urobilinogen - one of the chemicals routinely tested on urinalysis that when positive can indicate liver disease.

urgency – a sudden desire to urinate.

Urolift - a minimally invasive procedure for lower urinary tract symptoms due to blockage by the prostate.

varicocoele - a dilation of the veins in the scrotum that drain the testes, frequently described as a mass of varicose veins in the scrotum or "bag of worms."

vas deferens/vas – a thin tube about the diameter of a piece of spaghetti that carries sperm from the epididymis in the scrotum to the prostate where it meets the seminal vesicles to form the ejaculatory duct.

vasovasostomy - a procedure that attaches (anastomoses) two ends of the vas deferens that have been previously separated due to a vasectomy.

VED (vacuum erection device) - a hollow plastic tube that fits over the penis. A pump (either mechanical or battery powered) is applied to the tube via a plastic hose to produce a vacuum and thus an erection, which is help up by a rubber band placed around the base of the penis.

virus - a 'bug' that cannot be seen under standard light microscopy because it's too small and that consists of a segment of DNA or RNA and a protein coat that is able to cause an infection by multiplying only within living cells of a host.

watchful waiting - specific to prostate cancer, it's observing a patient's untreated condition, applied when the risks of treatment far outweigh the benefits.

Xiaflex - a prescription medication (collagenase) used to treat Peyronie's Disease by injecting the medication directly into the plaque of the tunica albuginea (should be done only by a urologist).

REFERENCES

Introduction

Grad, Roland, et al. (2017) "Shared Decision Making in Preventative Medicine." PubMed Central, *Canadian Fam Physician*, Sept; 63(9):682-684 < https://www.ncbi.nlm.nih.gov/pmc/articles/PMC5597010//.

Elwyn, Gllyn, et al. (2012) "Shared Decision Making in Clinical Practice." *J Gen Intern Med*. Oct; 27(10):1361-1376 < https://www.ncbi.nlm.nih.gov/pmc/articles/PMC3445676/.

Chapter 1: Your Body s Plumbing

Kelly, Christopher and Landman, Jaimie (2012) *The Netter Collection of Medical Illustrations: Urinary System. Vol. 5, 2nd Edition*. Saunders Press.

Chapter 2: Mysteries of the Foreskin and Circumcision

Blank, Susan et. al, (2012) "Circumcision policy statement from American academy of pediatrics," *Pediatrics* 130 (3):585-586 < https://doi.org/10.1542/peds.2012-1989.

Gollaher, David L. (1994) "From ritual to science: The medical transformation of circumcision in America," *Journal of Social History* 28(1):5-36.

Larke NL, Thomas SL, dos Santos Silva I, Weiss HA. (2011) "Male circumcision and penile cancer: a systematic review and meta-analysis," *Cancer Causes Control.* Aug; 22(8):1097-110. doi: 10.1007/s10552-011-9785-9. Epub 2011 Jun 22. PMID: 21695385; PMCID: PMC3139859.

Prodger, J.L., Kaul, R. (2017) "The biology of how circumcision reduces HIV susceptibility: broader implications for the prevention field," *AIDS Res Ther* 14(49), https://doi.org/10.1186/s12981-017-0167-6.

Dunsmuir WD, Gordon EM. (1999) "The history of circumcision," *BJU Int* 83(1): 1-12.

Chapter 3: I'm Peeing Blood!

Loo R.K., Lieberman S.F., Slezak J.M. et al. (2013) "Stratifying risk of urinary tract malignant tumors in patients with asymptomatic microscopic hematuria," *Mayo Clin Proc* 88:129.

Barocas, Daniel, et al. (2020) "Microhematuria: AUA/SUFU Guideline," *Journal of Urology* Oct 1:778-786 < https://www.auajournals.org/doi/10.1097/JU.0000000000001297.

Chapter 4: Urinary Tract Infections

Blandy, John (1989) *Kidney and urinary infection, in: Lecture notes on urology, 4th ed.* London:Blackwell Scientific Publications, pp. 63-78.

Farrell K, et. al. (2021) "Treatment of uncomplicated UTI in males: a systematic review of the literature," *BJGP* Open. Apr 26; 5(2)<https://www.ncbi.nlm.nih.gov/pmc/articles/PMC8170603/.

Brusch, JL, et al. (2021) "Urinary tract infection (UTI) in males treatment and management," *Medscape* Jan <https://emedicine.medscape.com/article/231574-treatment#:~:text=Adult%20males%20with%20UTI%20should,symptom%20of%20dysuria%20with%20phenazopyridine.

Davis, NG and Silberman, M. (2022) *Bacterial Acute Prostatitis*. National Library of Medicine. July < https://www.ncbi.nlm.nih.gov/books/NBK459257/.

Chapter 5: Can't Pee, See Me

Blandy, John (1989) *The prostate gland, In: Lecture notes on urology, 4th ed.* London: Blackwell Scientific Publications, pp. 214-240.

Lerner, Lori, et. al. (2021) "Management of lower urinary tract symptoms attributed to BPH: AUA GUIDELINE PART I - Initial workup and medical management," *J Urol*, Oct 206(4):806-817.

Elterman, DS. et. al. (2021) "Is it time to offer true minimally invasive treatments (TMIST) for BPH? – A review of office-based therapies and introduction of a new technology category," *The Canadian Journal of Urology*; April, 28(2), 10580-10583.

McVary, K., et. al. (2011) "Update on AUA guideline on the management of BPH," *J Urol*. May 185:1793-1803.

Foster, H., et. al. (2019) "Surgical management of lower urinary tract symptoms attributed to BPH: AUA Guideline Amendment," *J Urol*. Sept 202(3):592-598.

Chapter 6: Should I Get a PSA?

Kearns, JT, et. al. (2018) "PSA screening, prostate biopsy, and treatment of prostate cancer in the years surrounding the USPSTF recommendation against prostate cancer screening," *Cancer*, May 124(I 13):2733-2739.

Carroll, Peter R., et al. (2016) "NCCN guidelines insights: prostate cancer early detection, version 2.2016," *Journal of the National Comprehensive Cancer Network* 14.5:509-519.

Jiang, C., Fedewa, S.A., Wen, Y., Jemal, A. and Han, X. (2021) "Shared decision making and prostate-specific antigen based prostate cancer screening following the 2018 update of USPSTF screening guideline," *Prostate Cancer and Prostatic Diseases*, 24(1):77-80.

Grossman, David C., et al. (2018) "Screening for prostate cancer: US Preventive Services Task Force recommendation statement," *JAMA* 319.18:1901-1913.

Barry, Michael J., and Joel B. Nelson. (2015) "Patients present with more advanced prostate cancer since the USPSTF screening recommendations," *The Journal of Urology* 194.6:1534-1536.

Carroll, P.H. and Mohler, J.L. (2018) "NCCN guidelines updates: prostate cancer and prostate cancer early detection," *Journal of the National Comprehensive Cancer Network*, 16(5S):620-623.

Van Poppel, H., Hogenhout, R., Albers, P., et al. (2021) "A European model for an organised risk-stratified early detection programme for prostate cancer," *European Urology Oncology*, 4(5):731-739.

Chapter 7: Prostate Cancer

Lieberman, S.F. (2014) *Prostate Cancer Action Plan: Choosing the Treatment That's Right for You. 1st Edition*, 2015 The Permanente Federation, LLC Adapted from the video Prostate Cancer Action Plan: by Stephen Lieberman, M.D., Stephen Lieberman, M.D.< https://kpactionplans.org/prostate-cancer/img/Prostate-Cancer_booklet.pdf

Lieberman S.F., Lam J, Williams S, Chen A, Presti J. (2020) *Prostate Cancer Action Plan: Choosing the Treatment That's Right for You 2nd Edition*, revised upon special commission of The Permanente Federation, LLC < https://kpactionplans.org/prostate-cancer/img/ProstateCancer_booklet.pdf (see reference list pp 60-63).

Chapter 8: Your Scrotum and Testicles

Wampler, S.M. and Llanes, M. (2010) "Common scrotal and testicular problems," *Primary Care: Clinics in Office Practice*, 37(3):613-626.

Khatri, G., Bhosale, P.R., Robbins, J.B., et al. (2022) „ACR Appropriateness Criteria® Newly Diagnosed Palpable Scrotal Abnormality," *Journal of the American College of Radiology*, 19(5):S114-S120.

Trivedi, H.M., Singla, N., Lafin, J., et al. (2020) "First Do No Harm: A Cautious, Risk-adapted Approach to Testicular Cancer Patients," *Reviews in Urology* 22(2):85.

Bourke, M.M. and Silverberg, J.Z. (2019) "Acute scrotal emergencies," *Emergency Medicine Clinics*, 37(4):593-610.

Cheng, L., Albers, P., Berney, D.M., et al. (2018) "Testicular cancer," *Nature Reviews Disease Primers*, 4(1):1-24.

Albers, P., Albrecht, W., Algaba, F., et al. (2015) "Guidelines on testicular cancer: 2015 update," *European Urology*, 68(6):1054-1068.

Stephenson, A., Eggener, S.E., Bass, E.B., et al. (2019) "Diagnosis and treatment of early stage testicular cancer: AUA guideline," *The Journal of Urology*, 202(2):272-281.

Chapter 9: Bladder Cancer

Lenis, A.T., Lec, P.M. and Chamie, K. (2020) "Bladder cancer: a review," *JAMA*, 324(19):1980-1991.

Chang, S.S., Boorjian, S.A., Chou, R., et al. (2016) "Diagnosis and treatment of non-muscle invasive bladder cancer: AUA/SUO guideline," *The Journal of Urology*, 196(4):1021-1029.

Ritch, C.R., et al. (2020) "Use and validation of the AUA/SUO risk grouping for nonmuscle invasive bladder cancer in a contemporary cohort," *The Journal of Urology*, 203(3):505-511.

Taylor, J., Becher, E. and Steinberg, G.D. (2020) Update on the guideline of guidelines: non-muscle-invasive bladder cancer. *BJU international*, 125(2):197-205.

Chang, S.S., et al. (2017) "Treatment of non-metastatic muscle-invasive bladder cancer: AUA/ASCO/ASTRO/SUO guideline," *The Journal of Urology, 198*(3):552-559.

Sathianathen, N.J., et al. (2019) "Robotic assisted radical cystectomy vs open radical cystectomy: systematic review and meta-analysis," *The Journal of Urology, 201*(4):715-720.

Hautmann, R.E., et al. (2015) "Urinary diversion: how experts divert," *Urology, 85*(1):233-238.

Daneshmand, S. et al. (2018) "Efficacy and Safety of Blue Light Flexible Cystoscopy with Hexaminolevulinate in the Surveillance of Bladder Cancer: A Phase III, Comparative, Multicenter Study" *The Journal of Urology 195* (5):1158-1165

Chu, C. et al (2021) "Use of Cxbladder Monitor during the COVID-19 Pandemic to reduce the frequency of surveillance cystoscopy" *The Journal of Urology 206* (3):1142e

Chapter 10:   Everybody Must Get Stones

Thakore, Plalak and Liang, Terrence (2022) *Urolithiasis*, National Library of Medicine, June < https://www.ncbi.nlm.nih.gov/books/NBK559101/.

Türk, C., et al. (2011) *Guidelines on urolithiasis*. European Association of Urology.

Trinchieri, A. (2008) "Epidemiology of urolithiasis: an update," *Clinical cases in mineral and bone metabolism, 5*(2):101.

Pradère, B., et al. (2018) "Evaluation of guidelines for surgical management of urolithiasis," *The Journal of Urology, 199*(5):1267-1271.

Strohmaier, W.L. (2016) *Recent advances in understanding and managing urolithiasis*. F1000Research, 5.

Chapter 11: Kidney Tumors, Cysts, and Masses

Israel, G.M. and Bosniak, M.A. (2005) "How I do it: evaluating renal masses," *Radiology*, 236(2):441-450.

Volpe, A., Cadeddu, J.A., Cestari, A., et al. (2011) "Contemporary management of small renal masses," *European Urology*, 60(3):501-515.

Campbell, S.C., Clark, P.E., Chang, S.S., et al. (2021) "Renal mass and localized renal cancer: evaluation, management, and follow-up: AUA guideline: part I," *The Journal of Urology*, 206(2):199-208.

Campbell, S.C., Uzzo, R.G., Karam, J.A., et al. (2021) "Renal mass and localized renal cancer: evaluation, management, and follow-up: AUA guideline: Part II," *The Journal of Urology*, 206(2):209-218.

Chapter 12:   Erectile Dysfunction

Bodie, J.A., Beeman, W.W. and Monga, M. (2003) "Psychogenic erectile dysfunction," *The International Journal of Psychiatry in Medicine*, 33(3):273-293.

McMahon, C.G. (2014) "Erectile dysfunction," *Internal Medicine Journal*, 44(1):18-26.

Heidelbaugh, J.J. (2010) "Management of erectile dysfunction," *American Family Physician*, 81(3):305-312.

Zou, Z., Lin, H., Zhang, Y. and Wang, R. (2019) "The role of nocturnal penile tumescence and rigidity (NPTR) monitoring in the diagnosis of psychogenic erectile dysfunction: a review," *Sexual Medicine Reviews*, 7(3):442-454.

Beckman, T.J., Abu-Lebdeh, H.S. and Mynderse, L.A. (2006) "Evaluation and medical management of erectile dysfunction," In *Mayo Clinic Proceedings* 81(3):385-390.

Shindel, A.W. and Lue, T. F. (2022) *Medical and surgical therapy of erectile dysfunction.* Available online at: Medical and Surgical Therapy of Erectile Dysfunction - Endotext - NCBI Bookshelf (nih.gov).

Chapter 13: Vasectomy

Weiske, W.H. (2001) "Vasectomy," *Andrologia*, 33(3):125-134.

Schwingl, P.J. and Guess, H.A. (2000) "Safety and effectiveness of vasectomy," *Fertility and sterility*, 73(5):923-936.

Awsare, N.S., Krishnan, J., Boustead, G.B., et al. (2005) "Complications of vasectomy," *Annals of the Royal College of Surgeons of England*, 87(6):406.

Barone, M.A., Hutchinson, P.L., Johnson, et al. (2006) "Vasectomy in the United States," 2002. *The Journal of urology*, 176(1):232-236.

Silber, S.J. (1977) "Microscopic vasectomy reversal," *Fertility and Sterility*, 28(11):1191-1202.

Li, S., Goldstein, M., Zhu, J. and Huber, D. (1991) "The no-scalpel vasectomy," *The Journal of urology*, 145(2):341-344.

Chapter 14: Emergencies and Trauma

Ludvigson, A.E. and Beaule, L.T. (2016) "Urologic emergencies," *Surgical Clinics*, 96(3):407-424.

Manjunath, A.S. and Hofer, M.D. (2018) "Urologic emergencies," *Medical Clinics*, 102(2):373-385.

Rosenstein, D. and McAninch, J.W. (2004) "Urologic emergencies," *Medical Clinics*, 88(2):495-518.

Davis, NF, et. al. (2016) "Incidence, cost, complications and clinical outcomes of iatrogenic urethral catheterization injuries: A prospective multi-institutional study," *J Urol.* Nov 196(5): 1473-1477.

ACKNOWLEDGEMENTS

This book took eight years to write. I relied on professional writers, teachers, colleagues, and friends to help with this process. Without their encouragement and expertise there would still be a disorganized mess of a file on my laptop. It is here that I would like to express my heartfelt gratitude to: Dr. Janice Harper, superb copywriter and editor, Dr. Roger Porter, English professor, author, food critic, and friend, Martin Stabler; the late Luis Halpert, M.D., John Barry, M.D., Rich Steinberg, M.D., Ron Loo, M.D., Jerry Slepack, M.D., Steven Skoog, M.D., P.J. Chandhoke, M.D., Doug Ackerman, M.D., Jeffrey Johnson, M.D., Patrick Maginn, M.D., Eugene Fuchs, M.D., the late Thomas Hatch, M.D., Roger Wicklund, M.D., Adriene Carmack, M.D., Craig Sadur, M.D., Thomas Kelsey, M.D., Matt Forsyth, M.D., Richard Burt, M.D., Matti Totonchy, M.D., Bruce Lowe, M.D., Ron Potts, M.D., LoAn Nguyen MD, Barbara Loeb, Jill Einstein, M.D., Keith Bachman, M.D., Christopher Nelson, M.D., Anita Nelson, Steve Williams, M.D., Violeta Rabrinovitch, Tim Carey, M.D., Avery Seifert, M.D., Tracy Sanford, John Scott, and Lyman Flayhive, and all of the M.A.V.E.N. Project volunteer specialists who provide specialty consultation to primary care providers and patients in over 200 free clinics in 19 U.S. States. I would also like to thank the over 50 Oregon

Health Science University residents whom I had the honor of sharing the joys of being a urologist with for 31 years. And, I thank my brother Lenny Lieberman, and sister Sherry Preiss.

Finally, special thanks to my wife Virginia, and my daughters Emily Karlberg (Lieberman), and Elizabeth Lieberman, M.D., who provided unconditional support throughout the eight years I worked on researching and writing this book.

INDEX

NOTES

[i] Belt E. Leonardo the Florentine (1452–1519). Invest Urol 1965;3:1–9.

[ii] Reprinted with permission from Barry MJ et al. *J Urol.* 1992;148:1549–1557.

[iii] See A review of the use of tadalafil in the treatment of benign prostatic hyperplasia in men with and without erectile dysfunction - PMC (nih.gov)

[iv] See Beta-sitosterols for benign prostatic hyperplasia - PubMed (nih.gov)

[v] G. Mikaelian, M. Sojka, Authenticating Saw Palmetto extract: a new approach, *Nutraceutical Business & Technology*, 2009; 5; 24-27.

[vi] Serenoa repens for benign prostatic hyperplasia | Cochrane

[vii] Parts of this chapter have been based on *Prostate Cancer Action Plan 2.0: Choosing the Treatment That's Right for You*, (2020) Stephen Lieberman, M.D., John Lam, M.D., MBA, FACS, Stephen G. Williams, M.D., Alex Chen and Joseph Presti, M.D., FACS, Kaiser Pemanente.

[viii] https://www.cdc.gov/cancer/uscs/about/stat-bites/stat-bite-prostate.htm

[ix] Immunotherapy has thus far been less effective for prostate cancer and in my view should be considered experimental therapy and reserved for those patients with metastatic disease.

[x] https://www.auajournals.org/doi/10.1097/JU.0000000000000475

[xi] In Portland there is a fairly large community of Ukrainians. For whatever reason, perhaps due to my ability to speak a little Russian, three of these Ukrainians (all men) were referred to see me for gross blood in their urine.

When I asked, "Where were you during the Chernobyl accident?" the answers were revealing. One drove a supply truck in and out of the accident site, the other two were downwind. All three were smokers. And all three had high grade bladder cancers. Eleven years after the accident, the incidence of bladder cancer in the region went from 26/100,000 to 36/100,000 https://www.ncbi.nlm.nih.gov/pmc/articles/PMC5926045/. Of course, this is a much more complicated discussion now almost 40 years after the accident, but the fact remains that the incidence of bladder cancer rose significantly among those exposed to the radiation.

[xii] It's actually more complicated than this with 12 different T stages ranging from Ta (a papillary tumor confined to the lining mucosa) to T4a and T4b (tumor has grown out of the bladder and is invading the abdominal wall, adjacent organs).

[xiii] https://pubs.rsna.org/doi/10.1148/radiol.14122908

[xiv] https://www.nature.com/articles/s41443-020-00365-9.

[xv] The list is long. https://www.mayoclinic.org/drugs-supplements/sildenafil-oral-route/side-effects/drg-20066989?p=1

[xvi] https://www.plannedparenthood.org/learn/birth-control/condom/how-effective-are-condoms.

Made in United States
Troutdale, OR
08/24/2024

22291679R00204